Monographs in Neonatology

Thomas K. Oliver, Jr., M.D.
Series Editor

ANTIMICROBIAL THERAPY FOR NEWBORNS:
PRACTICAL APPLICATION OF PHARMACOLOGY
TO CLINICAL USE
by George H. McCracken, Jr., M.D., and John D. Nelson, M.D.

TEMPERATURE REGULATION AND ENERGY
METABOLISM IN THE NEWBORN
Edited by John C. Sinclair, M.D.

HOST DEFENSES IN THE NEONATE
by Michael E. Miller, M.D.

PERINATAL COAGULATION
by William E. Hathaway, M.D., and John Bonnar, M.D.

NEONATAL HYPERBILIRUBINEMIA
by Gerard B. Odell, M.D.

NEONATAL NECROTIZING ENTEROCOLITIS
Edited by Edwin G. Brown, M.D., and Avron Y. Sweet, M.D.

RETROLENTAL FIBROPLASIA:
A MODERN PARABLE

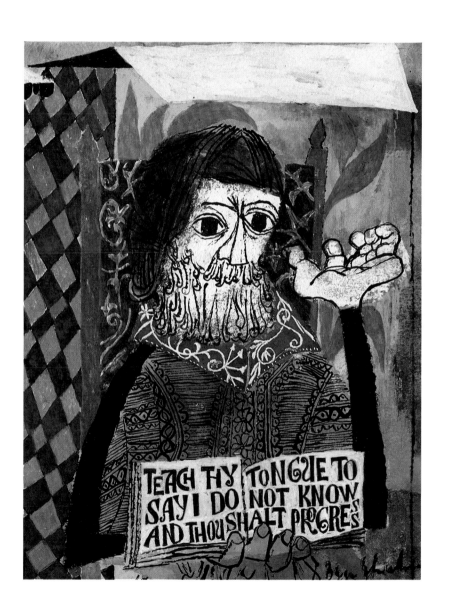

TEACH THY TONGUE TO SAY I DO NOT KNOW AND THOU SHALT PROGRESS

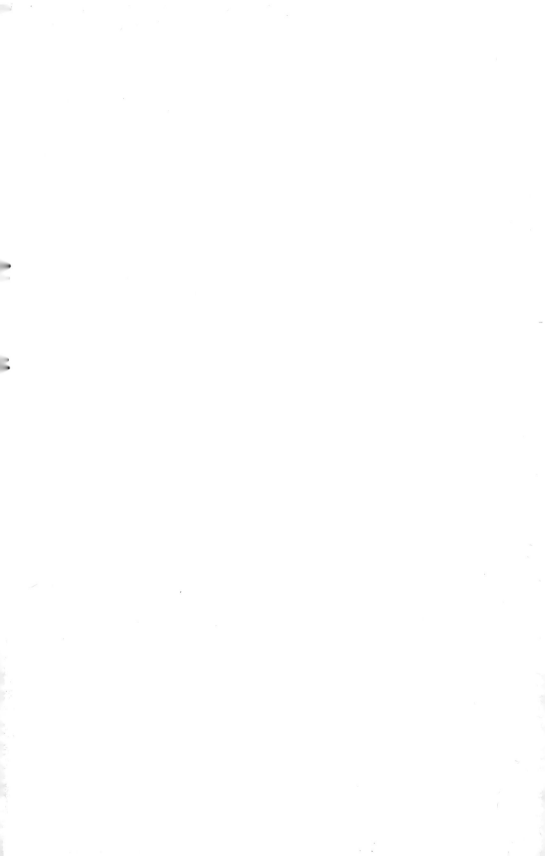

RETROLENTAL FIBROPLASIA: A MODERN PARABLE

William A. Silverman, M.D.
Formerly Professor of Pediatrics
College of Physicians and Surgeons
Columbia University
New York, New York

Grune & Stratton
A Subsidiary of Harcourt Brace Jovanovich, Publishers
NEW YORK   LONDON   TORONTO   SYDNEY   SAN FRANCISCO

The frontispiece was made possible by the friends and

admirers of William A. Silverman.

Library of Congress Cataloging in Publication Data

Silverman, William A
    Retrolental fibroplasia: A modern parable
    (Monographs in neonatology)
    Bibliography: p. 207
    Includes index.
    1. Retrolental fibroplasia. I. Title. [DNLM:
1. Retrolental fibroplasia. WW270 S587r]
RJ313.S54   362.1'9892011   80-11514
ISBN 0-8089-1264-X

Grune & Stratton, Inc.
111 Fifth Avenue
New York, New York 10003

Distributed in the United Kingdom by
Academic Press, Inc. (London) Ltd.
24/48 Oval Road, London NW 1

Library of Congress Catalog Number   80-11514
International Standard Book Number 0-8089-1264-X

Printed in the United States of America

This book is dedicated
to
Ruth

אשת חיל מי ימצא
ורחק מפנינים מכרה*

Contents

Figures

Tables

Acknowledgments

This book would still be waiting for "all the evidence to come in," if it were not for the urging of Dr. Robert W. Winters. For years I was at the water's edge, like Horace's rustic, waiting for the river to flow away before crossing. I was finally forced to take the plunge when Bob Winters asked me to inaugurate the Richard L. Day Lectureship at Columbia University in April 1975, and I could no longer delay recording the story of RLF about which I have talked so often in the past.

Over the years since the hectic period of the 1942–1954 RLF epidemic, I have corresponded with most of the protagonists in the disjointed struggle to overcome our ignorance about this disorder. More recently, I asked a number of the old campaigners to record their second thoughts, to recall unwritten incidents, and to set some parts of the printed record straight. They have been generous with long letters, tape recordings and telephone calls. I acknowledge their responses with warm gratitude, and hasten to absolve them of any responsibility for the way in which I have used the material which they provided. With few exceptions my confederates have agreed to allow me to send their letters and tape recordings to the National Library of Medicine, in Bethesda, Maryland, for deposit; future historians will deal with their contributions more fairly, I am sure, than I have in this account.

The dramatis personae—physicians, engineers, a nurse, an educator, a bioethicist, and a retired executive—who responded to my letters, from far and wide, are Christian B. Andreasen, Norman Ashton, J. D. Baum, Paul A. Chandler, Stewart H. Clifford, Harry Cullumbine, Richard L. Day, John T. Flynn, Gerald E. Gaull, Samuel Y. Gibbon, James L. Gillon, Harry H. Gordon, James R. Grosholz, Lars J. Gyllensten, Albert Jonsen, V. Everett Kinsey, Berthold Lowenfeld, Lula Lubchenco, Jerold F. Lucey, Rustin McIntosh, John B. McPherson, Arnall Patz, Priscilla Parke, Dale L. Phelps, Algernon B. Reese, and Clement A. Smith. I am indebted to many of these colleagues (and to their publishers) for allowing me to reproduce figures and tables from printed works (specific acknowledgments appear in the Notes and References section).

Librarian Julie Schmidt responded cheerfully to my endless demands on her time and talent; I am very grateful to her. Ellen Hirsch converted my tortured scribbling to a legible typescript with amazing accuracy and with loving devotion. Anne M. Schmid went over the text with a practiced eye and gave much good advice. The photographic wizardry of Steve Hubbard, the artistry of Leona Allison, and the graphic skill of Lee Romero earned my admiration and I thank them for their help.

It is impossible to acknowledge, adequately, the many contributions of my wife to this volume, and, most important to me, she never lost faith.

Foreword

It is a great delight to have this volume as part of the series, Monographs in Neonatology. The least important reason—though it is a terribly important one and a current problem in neonatal intensive care nurseries—is the major theme of the book, retrolental fibroplasia. As Dr. Silverman clearly indicates there are many, many aspects of this diesease that are not yet understood with respect to pathogenesis and prevention, though the major culprit, hyperoxia, has long since been identified.

A more important reason for welcoming the volume is that it is indeed a modern parable, and the lessons retrolental fibroplasia can teach us are important ones for us to learn today. Proper design of clinical investigative studies is often still woefully weak, and that which is declared as "evidence" frequently does not survive careful scrutiny.

But the most important reason for cheering this edition to the series is to have Bill Silverman again out front where he so rightfully belongs. If anyone can be described as the father of modern neonatal intensive care it surely is he. And even if doubting Thomases would care to challenge that statement, none would dare challenge the singular role he has had in advancing the cause of patient care by thoughtfully conceived and designed randomized controlled clinical trials. His scholarship in this arena is unrivaled in pediatrics.

As the Series Editor I salute both this volume and its author.

THOMAS K. OLIVER, JR., M.D.
SERIES EDITOR

Preface

Retrolental fibroplasia (RLF), a newly recognized disorder of premature infants, was described in 1942. After 12 years of bafflement and after thousands of babies were blinded, the outbreak was related to the use of supplemental oxygen in the first days of life. Soon after the mystery was "solved," I began to collect material on the epidemic with a thought to recording a history of this incredible experience. For more than 20 years, I related the RLF story to generations of interns and medical students. They responded with glazed-eye incomprehension, much as I had reacted at their age when I was told about infantile scurvy, a disease seen rarely in the modern era. In standard textbooks of pediatrics, RLF was dismissed, in very little space, as a curio. Throughout this period, I stubbornly insisted that the outbreak deserved study because it taught valuable lessons. Moreover, our understanding of the disorder itself, in terms of basic mechanisms, was still rudimentary. I felt like an old Turk among young fogies.

As time went on I became convinced that the unpleasant memory of the most dramatic epidemic of infantile blindness in recorded history was being repressed in the collective consciousness of medicine because it was too painful to recall. A remark attributed to Sir Ernst Chain, concerning another disaster in perinatal medicine, strengthened my suspicion. While agreeing that the thalidomide tragedy was of great significance to the people affected, Chain dismissed the whole affair as a chance occurrence—unfortunate but a random event and deserving no further attention. At the Congress of the Australian and New Zealand Association for the Advancement of Science in 1975, he was quoted as saying:

> . . . the [thalidomide story is] insignificant, it [has] been exaggerated out of all proportion and people should forget it.

I submit that we are completely irresponsible if we fail to make an attempt to understand how it came about that more than 10,000 children throughout the world were blinded as the result of a relatively minor change in caretaking practice! Moreover, the RLF incident was not an isolated occurrence. It foreshadowed, only too accurately, the shape of things to come (the thalidomide incident occurred after the RLF experience). In the dark words of the dramatist David Garrick:

> Prologues precede the piece—in mournful verse;
> As undertakers before the hearse.

When other treatment disasters followed on the heels of the blindness epidemic, I had a depressing sense of the déjà vu: I had been there before. And I must say, the odd sensation has returned frequently in the past few years as changes are being made more often and the therapies are more powerful than ever before. The need for review of the lessons of the recent past has become, in my opinion, urgent.

In the present volume, I present an interpretive history of the rise and fall of RLF, and I recount a number of similar tragedies which occurred in the years following the blindness outbreak. This look-back provides some insights into a general problem: the knotty difficulties which arise between the time when a new treatment is proposed and the time when the innovation is accepted by physicians for everyday care. I do not propose that error can be eliminated during this process, but I will argue, in the pages which follow, that the *extent* of medical disasters caused by inevitable missteps can be contained.

My focus, in reviewing the record of the past, centers on two areas of concern: (1) weaknesses in methodology, i.e., wasteful strategies for problem-solving in clinical medicine; and (2) the widening disagreement about goals, which has come to separate the medical community from the community-at-large.

The nature of my concern about the first matter is seen in how the problem of RLF arose and how it was "solved." The following incident is revealing. When I finished a draft of the early history of the blindness disaster in preparation for the Day Lectures at Columbia University in 1975, I sent it to a leading figure in American pediatrics. In return, I received a brusque note which read, "You have an interesting story to tell, but tell it right!" One sentence in my draft had upset him. This followed an account of the first two examples of RLF in Boston and read: "From these vague beginnings a giant iatrogenic episode was to evolve." My confrere felt that listeners would conclude from my words that the RLF epidemic had been "made in Boston." (In fact, RLF was called the "Boston disease" during the early years of the epidemic.) I amended the offending sentence for the talks in New York, but I could not put this exchange out of my mind.

After some thought, I came to the conclusion that the tragedy was, indeed, "made" in Boston, in New York, in Baltimore and in other teaching and research centers throughout the world. The RLF catastrophe would not have been extensive if pediatric leaders had insisted that scientific rules of evidence must be satisfied before any new technique in management of premature infants was used in teaching centers.

Although this hindsight seems simple-minded, surprisingly, little has changed. The scientific method is still honored only with lip reverence by most leaders in present-day clinical medicine. Moreover, their actions are not lost on students and trainees who will determine future action; most have concluded that strict rules of evidence can be set aside in dealing with the assessment of a new treatment for patients.

My second area of emphasis is summed up in a recent remark by a nurse to a group of RLF-blinded young adults. In a discussion of the dilemmas which confront caretakers in present-day intensive care nurseries when oxygen must be administered to keep very small premature infants alive, she said, "When I go home after work, I find myself asking, 'Am I doing it [making heroic technologic efforts] for you or for me'?" Her question should be pondered by all thoughtful citizens. There is some indication that the community-at-large is having second thoughts about medicine's headlong rush into the brave new world. And, I must add, physicians are tossing in their beds more fitfully than in the past.

My account is not addressed primarily to experienced neonatologists and perinatologists. As a result, I have made a conscious attempt to avoid innundating nonconversant readers with a flood of technical details about RLF, respiratory distress syndrome, kernicterus, etc. Some of the detail will be found in the Notes and References section for each chapter, and readers are directed to published citations for complete descriptions of evidence. (The citations are arranged alphabetically, by author, in the Bibliography section.)

Since I firmly believe that we learn from our mistakes, I have gone to great lengths to point out the errors of the past. My chronicle, therefore, is not a balanced account of the accomplishments in perinatal medicine. However, there has been no dearth of praise by others for the achievements in this new field. Most of the plaudits are well deserved. Indeed, the pediatric research establishment, suffering from severe reductions in public funds for research, has mounted public-relations-guided self-congratulatory efforts; one was entitled, ''Voyages to Discovery.'' My tale dwells on the shipwrecks during these voyages.

The critical tone which I have adopted in this book may try the readers' patience. I do hope they will keep before them the advice of Karl Popper:

> . . . if we respect truth, we must search for it by persistently searching for our errors, by indefatigable rational criticism and self-criticism.

RETROLENTAL FIBROPLASIA:
A MODERN PARABLE

1

A New Affliction In Premature Infants

On February 14, 1941, Doctor Stewart H. Clifford, a Boston pediatrician, made a routine home visit to examine an infant girl born prematurely the previous November. Doctor Clifford remembers this house call as follows:

The father, I recall, was a young rabbi and the family lived . . . [at 2 Elm Hill Park, Roxbury]. Although the baby's general development was excellent, I was shocked to note roving nystagmus, and opacities in the eyes, and I had to tell the family I was afraid the baby could not see. I immediately referred the baby to one of our leading ophthalmologists, Doctor Paul [A.] Chandler.

Doctor Chandler examined the infant and made this note on his office record:

. . . shows a searching nystagmus of both eyes. Anterior chambers almost flat. Pupils react to light. Faint red reflex above, but below there is a grayish reflex.

He told Doctor Clifford he had not seen anything like it before, and arranged an admission to the Massachusetts Eye and Ear Infirmary for examination under ether and for consultation with Doctor Frederick Verhoeff, one of the period's leading authorities in eye pathology. The examination, carried out on February 19, 1941, revealed a grayish membrane covered with blood vessels which appeared to be on the back surface of the

1

lens of both eyes. A descriptive label, "fibro-vascular sheath of the lens," was applied to the unusual condition. An operation was considered but dismissed because Doctor Verhoeff thought the outlook was so poor.

In the meantime, on a Sunday afternoon in the same month, Doctor Clifford received an urgent call from a prominent Boston family asking him to examine a twin infant who had been born on July 13, 1940, weighing 1.02 kg (2 lb 4 oz) at delivery; the co-twin had not survived. Doctor Clifford recalls:

> I went to the family apartment on Beacon Street to find there had been a family gathering with the Philadelphia members of the family, and one of the relatives noted the eyes of the infant boy [now 7 months old] were behaving strangely. When I arrived I was shocked to find my second case within a week of my first. I told them [the family] of my suspicions and of my previous case. They wanted immediate action, so I called Doctor Chandler—he was out of town. I called Trigve Gunderson—he was away. I finally got hold of Doctor [Theodore] Terry.
>
> Terry soon arrived with all of his equipment and declared that the condition was congenital cataracts. He arranged for admission to Children's Hospital the next day for operation. I insisted that both Doctors Chandler and Verhoeff be called in consultation prior to any operation. This was done and we all gathered in the operating room amphitheatre at the Children's. They were able to convince Doctor Terry that the condition was not operable.

Doctor Chandler's memory of that interesting morning is as follows:

> The day after I saw the first case, I happened to walk by the operating room door and Doctor Terry asked me to come in and look at a baby on whom he was about to operate for what he thought was a congenital cataract. Fresh from the experience of the day before, I recognized that this was the same thing, and of course, no operation was done.

Boston Lying-In Hospital has preserved the nursery records of these two children who were the first to be diagnosed as afflicted by what came to be called "retrolental fibroplasia" (literally, scar tissue behind the lens of the eye). The neologism was coined in 1944 by Doctor Harry Messenger of Boston, an ophthalmologist who was also a Latin and Greek scholar.

The scion had been delivered by Doctor Frederick Irving on July 13, 1940, the first born of twins and, as noted, he weighed 1.02 kg (2 lb 4 oz). The fetal membranes had ruptured 4 days earlier, and the placenta and membranes showed signs of inflammation.

The co-twin was female and weighed 1.01 kg (2 lb 3½ oz). The fetal membranes were intact and there was no inflammation, but she had breathing difficulty and died at 6 hours of age. A diagnosis of "respiratory failure" was recorded (an autopsy was not performed).

The initial care prescribed for the surviving boy was typical for the time (Fig. 1-1). In describing the infant the nurses noted: "cries well" and "color good" (Fig. 1-2). The findings of physical examination were not recorded on the chart.

The rabbi's daughter was born on November 23, 1940; premature labor was brought on by an abnormally low position of the placenta in the uterus. Her birthweight was 1.81 kg (4 lb). After a physical examination the baby was described as "O.K.," and the nurses' notes indicated that the infant's condition was good. The initial orders were "routine premi regime", which included the same measures used for the first infant (Fig. 1-1). On the second and third days of life there were several spells of cyanosis, but no other difficulties were recorded.

The two Boston infants were the forerunners of an epidemic of blindness which rose to unsurpassed heights throughout the world in the next twelve years. In 1942, Terry published a brief note describing the unique eye condition of the Beacon Hill twin and noted the following:

> One of the consultants, Doctor Paul A. Chandler, has a case almost identical in appearance, in an infant also born prematurely . . . Recently three other cases have been seen in the clinic of the Massachusetts Eye and Ear Infirmary . . .

Terry went on to speculate about mechanisms to explain this odd affliction. Finally, he wrote two prophetic sentences in the first announcement of the disorder:

> In view of these findings [all 5 instances occurred in infants born prematurely] perhaps this complication should be expected in a certain percentage of premature infants. If so, some new factor has arisen in extreme prematurity to produce such a condition.

Between 1942 and 1945 Terry collected 117 examples of the new type of blindness. He became convinced the condition developed following birth because in three prematurely born infants whose eyes were normal after delivery, he subsequently found well-established retrolental fibroplasia (RLF). Before his death in 1946, Terry made extensive studies on the development and regression of the fetal blood vessels of the eye and attempted, without success, to reproduce the disease via experiments in young opossums and rats.

Despite Terry's observation that the eyes of some RLF victims were normal at birth, the notion persisted among physicians until 1948 that there was either an inherent or acquired abnormality of the eye caused by factors which operated before birth or, at the latest, immediately thereafter.

In 1948, William and Ella Owens, husband-and-wife ophthalmolo-

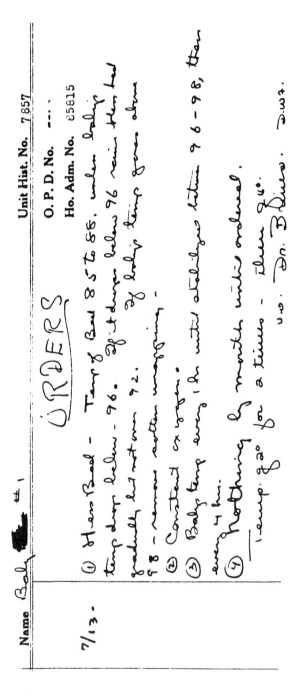

Fig. 1-1. Doctor's orders prescribing the initial care for the surviving twin infant boy born in Boston Lying-In Hospital on July 13, 1940. The orders read as follows:

"1. Hess Bed [see Fig. 7-1]—Temp of Bed 85 to 88[°F]. Unless baby's temp drops below 96. If it drops below 96 raise [temperature of] Hess Bed gradually but not over 92. If baby's temp goes above 98—remove cotton wrapping.

2. Constant oxygen [piped into bed from an oxygen tank beside the bed— see Fig. 7-1].

3. Baby's temp every 1 h until stabilized between 96–98, then every 4 hrs.

4. Nothing by mouth until ordered. Temp q 2° [hours] for 2 times—then q 4° V.O. [vocal order] Dr. Brines. D.W.F. [nurse's initials]"

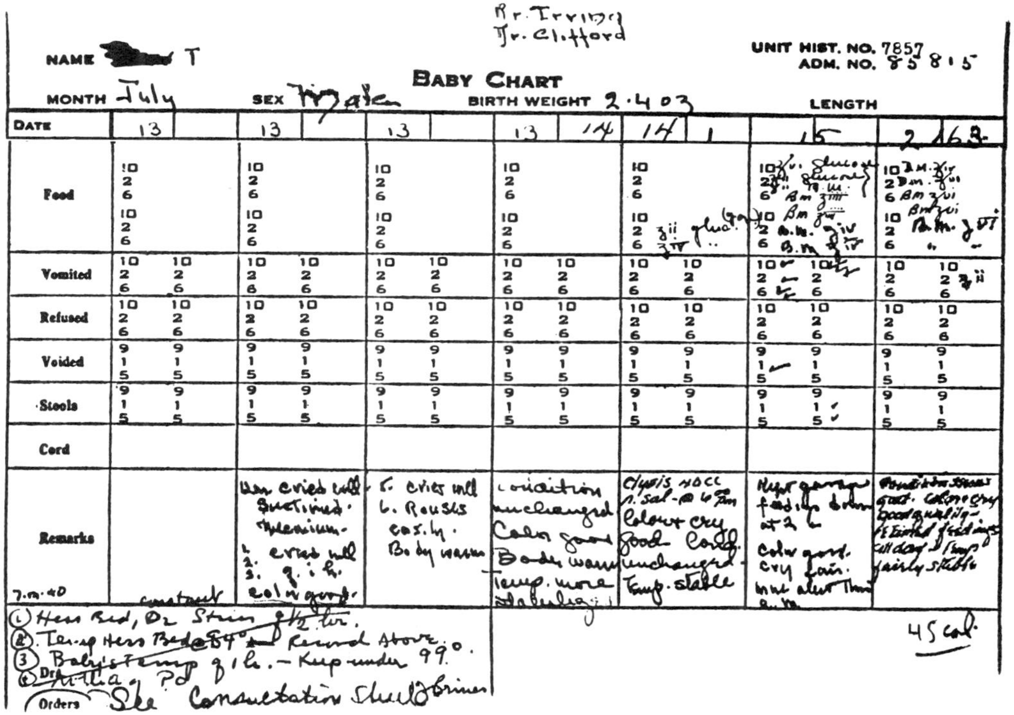
NAME [redacted] T
BABY CHART
UNIT HIST. NO. 7857
ADM. NO. 85815
MONTH July
SEX Male
BIRTH WEIGHT 2.403
LENGTH
DATE
Food
Vomited
Refused
Voided
Stools
Cord
Remarks
Orders

Fig. 1.2 Hospital chart recording the events of the first 4 days of life in the surviving twin infant boy (see Fig. 1-1). The nurse's summarize the doctor's orders (lower left panel). The initial "Remarks" on admission to the nursery read:

"12 n [noon] cried well-
Suctioned-
Meconium-
1. Cried well
2. q [every] i h [hour]
3. Color good."

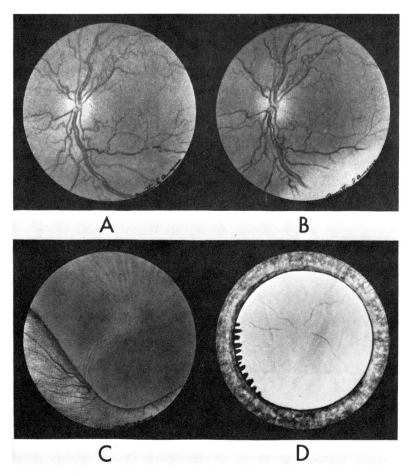

Fig. 1-3. The development of RLF described by Owens and Owens in 1948 (appearance of the retina through a direct ophthalmoscope). A. An early stage showing dilated and tortuous blood vessels of the retina. B. Later stage, showing an elevation of the retina developing in the periphery of the eye. C. Further extension of the elevated retina, appearing as a membrane at the edge of the retinal field. D. Complete retrolental membrane, with blood vessels coursing over the completely separated retina. At this stage the pupil appears white. (For a description of the early changes seen with modern equipment see Fig. 9-1.)

gists at the Wilmer Ophthalmological Institute of Johns Hopkins Hospital and University, examined more than 200 premature infants at birth by direct inspection of the interior of the eyes with an opthalmoscope; none had RLF. Half of these babies were patiently examined at monthly intervals until the age of 6 months; 4 percent developed RLF. They described the progressive development of changes in the ophthalmoscopic appearance of the blood vessels of the retina, beginning at 2½ to 3½ months after birth.

As depicted in Figure 1-3, the first detectable abnormality was slight enlargement of the caliber of arteries and veins in the retina. The size of the vessels increased, the orderly course of the arteries and veins became convoluted, and soon the retina itself became elevated in the far peripheral regions of the eye. Grayish masses of detaching retinal tissue increased in size and extent and, after a short time, a gray membrane (the detached retina covered with many enlarged blood vessels) billowed forward in the chamber of the eye and formed an opaque cast behind the lens. At this stage of the abnormal process, the pupils of the eye appeared white even to an untrained observer (Fig. 1-4). Both eyes were usually involved and, not infrequently, the severity of the changes was unequal.

These observations, which made early diagnosis possible, were confirmed rapidly. It soon became routine in many large research hospitals throughout the world to examine the interior of the eyes of the premature infants at weekly intervals. By the end of the 1940s, the dimensions of the RLF epidemic were becoming evident. The startling new complication alarmed all who were making efforts to preserve the lives of premature infants and many now paused to review the development of special procedures in newborn care, in the hope of detecting a clue to this mystery.

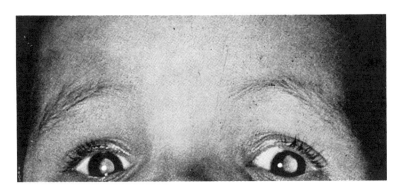

Fig. 1-4. End stage of RLF with completely detached retinas presenting as white membranes filling the pupil of the eye. The child is totally blind.

2

The Evolvement of Care for Feeble and Prematurely Born Infants

Humankind is not exempt from the general biologic rule of reproductive extravagance. In all species of living creatures, the number of individuals who survive the fetal period, birth, and early infancy has been, throughout millenia, only a small fraction of the total number of beings launched at conception. Humanity's place within the balance of competing species was maintained by high rates of reproduction and by attentive nurturing of newborn infants who are immature and dependent as compared with the precocious status of the newborn of many other mammals. Without elaborate techniques of hygiene and supportive care, relatively few human infants can survive the immediate newborn period or the first months of infancy. The toll of life has always been disproportionately high among the smallest, most enfeebled offspring, i.e., those born prematurely or those who are small and weak because of retarded growth or maldevelopment.

However, the concept that these "expected losses" should be prevented is a relatively new idea in human history. Harris presents evidence which suggests that our stone-age ancestors experienced reproductive pressures and consequent environmental depletions which led to the practice of infanticide. He concludes that this strategy (especially the killing of female infants to reduce reproductive potential) was used regularly by prehistoric cultures in order to keep their populations low in relation to the means of subsistence. Infanticide was also practiced by many civilizations; for example, in Roman Law the father of the family was bidden to destroy deformed children. the stabilization of population in Japan between 1726 and 1852 has been attributed to widespread infanticide (the practice was called "mabiki", literally "thinning out"). McKeown has adduced that the modern rise of population is due, in no small part, to the decrease of infanticide in most areas of the world.

Even when rescue of less-than-robust infants was seen as a desirable social goal, the first life-support efforts were halting and crude. In some ancient societies, weak newborn infants were wrapped in wadding or sheep skin, with the wool adhering, to protect them from excessive heat loss. The peasants of Silesia and Westphalia placed feeble infants in a jar full of feathers. In England, the cot or cradle was put close to the hearth, and the fire tended night and day to provide constant heat. Directions for the control of heat exchange between the delicate neonate and his environment are contained in an old quatrain:

> Thou, Nurse in swaddling Bands the Babe
>   enfold,
> And carefully defend its Limbs from
>   Cold:
> If Winter by the Chimney place thy
>   Chair
> If Summer, then admit the cooling Air . . .

In 1780, Chaussier experimented with the use of the newly discovered gas, oxygen, in newborn infants who failed to establish normal respirations. Meissner advised, in 1838, that premature and debilitated neonates be given enemas of human milk and two milk baths each day, in addition to oral feedings of mothers' milk. The first specially designed incubator, a double-walled heated tub for human infants, is attributed to von Rühl of St. Petersburg, Russia, in 1835; an identical device was described by Denucé of Bordeaux, France in 1857 (Fig. 2-1), and by Credé at the University of Leipzig in the early 1860s.

Concerted efforts to save infants began following the immense loss of life in France from military action and the months of famine during the seige of Paris in the Franco–Prussian War (1870–1871). In England, the steady fall of the birthrate, beginning in 1871, was cited as evidence for the need to conserve the lives of all infants, ". . . even the prematurely born . . .," for "economic as well as sentimental" reasons.

In 1878, E. S. Tarnier, a leading Parisian obstetrician, visited an

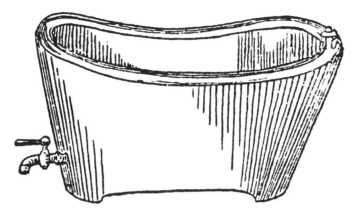

Fig. 2-1.   Warm tub with double-wall jacket first used by Denucé in 1857. Hot water was installed into the top petcock (right) and removed from the bottom spigot.

exhibition, the Jardin d'Acclimation, and came across a warming chamber for the rearing of poultry, devised by M. Odile Martin of the Paris Zoo. He asked Martin to build a similar box, sufficiently ventilated and large enough to hold one or two premature infants (Fig. 2-2). This was done and the first warm-air incubators were used at the Paris Maternité Hospital in 1880. In a report presented to the Academy of Medicine of France in 1895, the following note appeared:

> The minute and delicate care which these weakly [prematurely born] infants require, especially in winter, to protect them from the cold is so great that till now most of them have died . . . since Doctor Tarnier introduced . . . the ingenious contrivance, called a "couveuse," a large number of these infants have been saved.

In 1884, Tarnier began to use intragastric tube feedings of human milk (gavage) in the care of premature infants, a technique which was successful in supporting the nutrition of the smallest and most feeble infants who were unable to suck.

Winckel, in 1882, attempted to rear small infants in a womblike warm bath (Fig. 2-3), but the device was impractical and was not widely copied. On the other hand, a giant walk-in incubator (3.6 × 1.8 meters) for infants and their attendants, designed by Colerat in 1886, was imitated. Glassed-in, hot-air rooms were used for many years in a number of large hospitals in Europe and in the United States.

In 1888, Pierre Budin of Paris began to publish articles describing his experience at the Maternité Hospital with the care of premature infants.

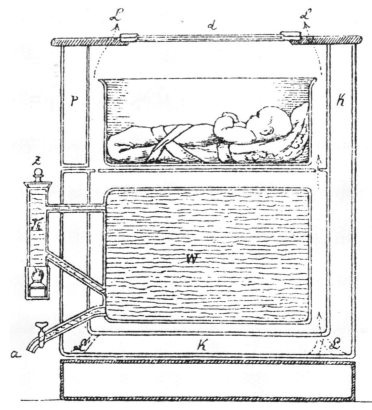

Fig. 2-2.   The Tarnier-Martin couveuse. A double-wall chamber (K) with a glass top (d) and a door (P) opening into the infant compartment. Warming was accomplished by heating water with an oil flame in an external "thermo-syphon" (Th) connected to a large water chamber (W) beneath the infant section. The closed incubator was ventilated by a rising current of warm air (L). Arrows indicate the flow of air from entry ports at the base of the unit, around the water chamber, to exit ports at the top of the baby compartment. Z indicates the opening for water fill; (a) was the emptying pet-cock.

Through the influence of Madame Henry, formerly chief midwife at this hospital, he established a special department for "weaklings" at the end of 1893. Budin also was appointed to the Clinique Tarnier in 1898 and, under his tutelage, these two hospitals in Paris became the first centers in the world for specialized studies of premature infant care. In ten lectures to his students, published in 1900, Budin enunciated three basic problems in care of the prematurely born:

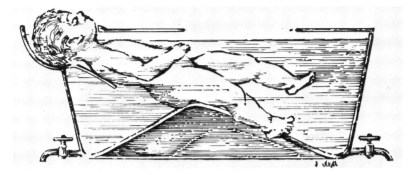

Fig. 2-3. Winckel's warming bath for premature infants, 1882.

"1.   Their temperature and their chilling;
 2.   Their feeding;
 3.   The diseases to which they are prone."

The Tarnier incubator (improved with a "Regnard regulator", a moni-toring device which activated an electric bell to warn against over-warming) was used at Charité by Budin to solve the thermal problem. He advocated human milk feedings to solve the second problem by nursing at the breast of mother, or wet nurses when possible. If the infant was unable to suckle, milk was hand-expressed in a trickle into his mouth, fed by spoon into the mouth (or into the nose by means of a special "nasal spoon"), or intro-duced directly into the stomach by intermittent gavage. Budin began the practice of weighing the infant before and after feeding to calculate the amount of milk taken in 24 hours by infants of different birth size. From this, he concluded that a premature infant should ". . . take, in general, a quantity of milk equal to or a little more than one-fifth of its body-weight" each day.

Proneness to infection was the risk stressed in the third of Budin's considerations. Following a severe epidemic of respiratory infections among premature infants at the Maternité Hospital in 1896, Budin became con-vinced of the importance of special precautions. In the same year, he proposed the following plan for a special unit:

1.   Grouping together the healthy premature infants;
2.   Isolating the sick and suspect infants;
3.   Separating wet nurses' babies from contact with the premature infants;
4.   Establishing a milk room where "sterilized" milk could be heated;
5.   Keeping the bottles of sterilized milk cool in summer in an ice chamber;

6. Providing a toilet and dressing room for wet nurses where they were to ". . . wash their hands and face and don an overall" before ministering to their premature infant charges.

These guidelines for the care and feeding of premature infants were adopted slowly and with very little modification throughout the Western world.

The spread of Budin's ideas was spurred on under very curious circumstances. He asked a young associate, Martin Couney, to exhibit the newly modified Tarnier incubator at the World Exposition in Berlin in 1896, and armed him with a letter of introduction to Professor Czerny, an illustrious obstetrician. Couney hit upon the idea of placing live premature infants in the exhibit incubators and asked Czerny's help to obtain the babies. Czerny sent him to Empress Augusta Victoria, the protectress of Berlin's Charity Hospital, who agreed readily, since the premature infants were considered to have very little chance of survival. Couney brought six incubators and an entourage of Budin's nurses to the exposition and named the exhibit "Kinderbrutanstalt". The notion of a "child hatchery" caught the imagination of the Berlin public. Soon there were ribald songs about the exhibit in the beer halls and night clubs, and Couney's infant exhibit, located in the amusement section next to the Congo Village and the Tyrolean Yodelers, became a huge success. Several "batches" of infants were reared at the show and, according to Couney, "there were no deaths".

The following year Couney organized a similar exhibit of the Paris methods of care in Earl's Court, London, at the Victorian Era Exhibition. This exhibit received favorable reports in a number of editorials in the respected medical journal, The Lancet, which commented on the need to adopt these new French techniques to reduce the large number of infant deaths in England due to premature births.

Following these two successful experiences, Martin Couney was launched on a colorful and life-long career. With Madame Louise Recht, a Budin-trained nurse, Couney traveled throughout the United States and the world organizing live premature infant shows at virtually every large exposition. These exhibits grew so in size, that in 1901 at the Pan-American Exposition in Buffalo, New York an imposing building was erected specially for Couney's show of the Budin techniques (Fig. 2-4). (The first incubators purchased by the Children's Hospital of Buffalo were those used in the Pan-American Exposition.) Two years later, in 1903, Couney settled in the United States and his exhibit, for which he charged a 25¢ admission fee, became a fixture at Coney Island every summer for the next four

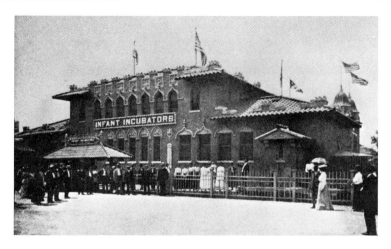

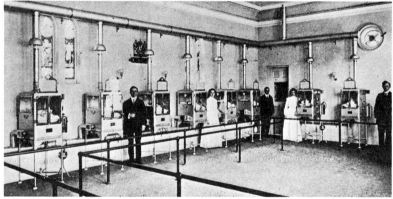

Fig. 2-4. The building and interior room with infant incubators for the demonstration–rearing of live premature infants at the Pan-American Exposition, Buffalo,
New York, 1901.

decades. Despite the bizarre side-show setting, he enjoyed a good reputa-
tion among obstetricians who referred babies to him for free care. His last
"Incubator Baby Exhibit" was in New York at the 1939 World's Fair.

Julius Hess organized the first conventional premature infant station
in the United States at the Sarah Morris Hospital, Chicago, in 1922. The
methods of care used by Hess and his chief nurse, Evelyn Lundeen, were
those developed by the French obstetricians and further popularized by
English and German physicians. Hess affirmed the influence of the show-
man Couney in the preface to his first textbook.

During the first four to five decades after the turn of this century, the care of prematurely born and feeble newborn infants became fairly routine. The results were judged satisfactory on the basis of hospital reports of a slow but steady rise in the survival rate of small neonates, although reliable national and international data were not collected until the late 1940s. The empirical techniques developed in Paris were rigidly applied by the expert nurses who ruled in premature units. Strict isolation measures discouraged traffic in the glass-enclosed rooms and parents had to observe their offspring from a distance; even physicians were discouraged from touching their charges too frequently.

This quiet, cloister-like atmosphere was shattered beyond recognition by the RLF epidemic. Soon after the widespread extent of the disorder was appreciated in the 1940s, it was noted with alarm that the complication seemed to occur most frequently in infants reared in premature infant nurseries with the most highly organized and advanced programs for care!

3
The First Decade of RLF

Terry's original guess that ". . . some new factor has arisen in extreme prematurity . . ." was supported by the retrospective studies of the Doctors Owens in Baltimore. They examined 128 children born between 1935 and 1944 and found no examples of RLF. There was only one instance of RLF (recognized in retrospect at age 16) among more than 200 carefully followed graduates of the Sarah Morris Premature Station in Chicago, born between the years 1922 and 1934. Other retrospective studies, principally by questionnaire, in eight large U.S. cities and in Birmingham, England, had disclosed only an occasional affected person before 1940. Algernon Reese surveyed the ophthalmologic reports published prior to 1944 and concluded that RLF occurred before Terry's report, but that it was rare.

The frequency of occurrence of RLF, first in the United States and later in other developed countries (including Canada, Britain, France, Sweden, Holland, Spain, Switzerland, Italy, Australia, Israel, Cuba, and South Africa) rose sharply at the end of the 1940s. By mid-century, RLF was regarded by ophthalmologists as the principal cause of blindness in infants. Although this opinion was based on incomplete surveys (Table 3-1 and Fig. 3-1) the epidemic of blindness was undeniable; by 1952, peculiar geographic and temporal variations were noted that could not be explained entirely by differences in reporting or in awareness of the condition by observers. The unfortunate preeminence of the "advanced" countries seemed to be explained by the fact that premature infant survival rates were highest

Table 3-1
The Four Most Frequent Causes of Blindness in
Preschool Children in Four States (1947)

Causes of Blindness	Illinois	New Jersey	New York	Wisconsin
Retrolental Fibroplasia	20	28	20	8
Cataract	9	18	15	14
Optic Atrophy	—	21	9	5
Glaucoma	3	10	11	—
...	⋮	⋮	⋮	⋮
Total	48	96	93	38

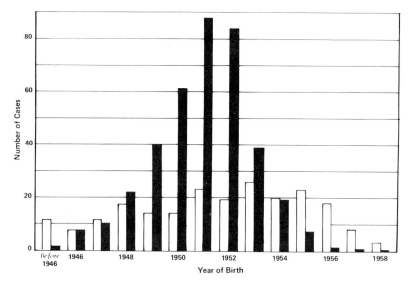

Fig. 3-1.   The field staff of the California School for the Blind found that RLF accounted for more than 80 percent of all cases of blindness in children born in Southern California during the years 1951–1952. (RLF is shown in solid bars, other causes of blindness in empty columns.)

in these parts of the world. More than 100 reports on RLF were published throughout the world in the three-year period 1950–1952 inclusive and over 50 separate "causes" were proposed (Appendix A). Approximately half of these factors were examined formally. Systematic sifting of evidence from experiences in the immediately preceding period established associations between RLF and 19 speculated "causes"; only five of these "causes" were tested by experimental (or quasi-experimental) planned clinical trials.

In 1949 Kinsey and Zacharias made the first attempt to seek an explanation for the increased frequency of RLF, by examining the concurrence of RLF and a number of factors relating to mothers and children (298 normal and 53 RLF-affected children) who were delivered in Boston Lying-In Hospital during the years 1938–1948. They found several associations:

1. The disorder occurred about half as often among first-born, when compared with subsequent birth-orders of premature infants.
2. ". . . infants in whom RLF subsequently developed, remained in the nursery water-jacketed incubator and in oxygen for longer periods than the infants in whom retrolental fibroplasia did not develop, suggesting that the general health of the infants in whom RLF developed may have been poorer than in those whose eyes remained normal or, possibly, that the latter were larger infants requiring a shorter stay in the hospital."
3. RLF occurred 1½ times more often in male than in female children.
4. Treatment of infants in the nursery changed in association with the annual percent occurrence of RLF. There was a correlation between increased blindness and (a) administration of iron, (b) the administration of a multiple water-miscible vitamin preparation, and (c) more frequent use of oxygen.

When these relationships were examined graphically (Fig. 3-2), it was found that "The correlation between the rise in incidence and dosage was less striking for oxygen than for water-miscible vitamin preparations and for iron."

The findings of this Boston survey with respect to vitamins and iron were of particular interest to the Baltimore ophthalmologists, Owens and Owens. It had been established in the early 1940s that prematurely born infants absorbed milk-fat inefficiently; artificial milk-mixtures (made with a relatively low concentrattion of fat and with a relatively high proportion of the mix as milk protein) appeared to overcome the absorptive handicap. Owens and Owens reasoned that the low-fat milk feedings would not supply premature infants with needed fat-soluble vitamins; and, since the requirement for these substances increased after birth, signs of deficiency would be expected to appear some weeks after delivery. They correlated this postulation with two observations: (1) the earliest changes of RLF *did*

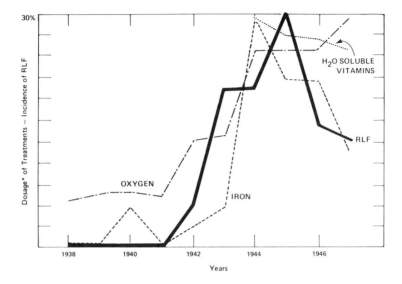

Fig. 3-2. Correlation between the frequency of RLF and three treatments in the premature nursery at the Boston Lying-In Hospital, 1938–1947; its occurrence tracked most closely with iron therapy (ferrous sulfate).
*Days in oxygen, drops of water-miscible vitamins, and drams of ferrous sulfate.

occur about one month after birth, and (2) only vitamin E, of all the fat-soluble vitamins, was not administered routinely to premature infants. In addition they took note of studies in experimental animals which indicated that the requirement of vitamin E increased when vitamin A was administered, and that iron salts destroyed vitamin E. The rise in frequency of RLF found by Kinsey and Zacharias in association with increased use of water-miscible preparations of vitamins (including vitamin A) and iron could be interpreted to indicate that the marginal vitamin E status of newborn premature infants was made worse by the newer treatments. All of these considerations, as well as arguments from studies of the biochemical functions of vitamin E, suggested that vitamin E supplements might prove effective in the treatment or prevention of RLF.

Beginning in 1949, Owens and Owens began to test their hypothesis. They administered a vitamin E preparation (alpha tocopherol acetate) to infants at the time the eyes showed early changes of RLF; the condition appeared to arrest in some infants. Following this experience, they undertook an experimental trial of vitamin E administered from birth. For a period of 10 months, alternate infants admitted to the premature nursery of Johns Hopkins Hospital were given either 150 mg a day of synthetic vitamin E, or no treatment. During this period 11 infants received vitamin E, none developed RLF; among 15 in the untreated control group, 5 developed RLF.

This early trend of difference was sufficient to impress Doctors Jonas Friedenwald and Alan Woods, leading ophthalmologists at Johns Hopkins Hospital. They persuaded the Doctors Owens to abandon the controlled trial. Subsequently all infants in the Baltimore nursery were given supplementary vitamin E by mouth. As word of this experience spread throughout the world, vitamin E prophylactic treatment to prevent RLF was started in many hospitals. The informal experience of nine other groups failed to confirm the Johns Hopkins experience, and the Doctors Owens were unable to demonstrate an impressive protective effect of vitamin E in the years following the aborted formal trial.

Although a decrease in severity did occur in prophylactically treated infants in Baltimore and in Boston, the quixotic temporal variability of the disease led most observers to doubt the significance of these trends. Additionally, no correlation could be found between blood levels of vitamin E and the occurrence of RLF. After a few years all interest in the vitamin E relationship to RLF had waned (see chapter notes).

Soon after a large premature center was opened in the fall of 1949 at Babies Hospital in New York City, my colleagues and I detected the first patient with RLF in this unit. My experience with this infant and subsequent events in New York are so revealing of the desperation felt by all who were faced with the mounting epidemic that it merits recounting. On February 15, 1950, Doctor Frederick Blodi, an ophthalmologist who had been examining the eyes of all infants in the new nursery at weekly intervals, made this note in the chart of an eight-week-old infant:

> Increased tortuosity of [retinal] veins!

One week later, February 21, there was no question in Doctor Blodi's mind and Doctor Algernon Reese agreed that the dilated and tortuous veins and diffuse hemorrhages in both eyes were the early signs of RLF.

This affected infant was the prematurely born daughter of a senior member of the Biochemistry Department of the College of Physicians and Surgeons at Columbia University. After six miscarriages, a pregnancy had proceeded to 29 weeks, and a 1.1 kg (2 lb 6 oz) girl was born. She was thriving at two months. The day following the detection of definite signs of RLF by Doctor Blodi, I wrote the following note in the chart:

Following the above-noted opinion [of Doctor Blodi] about the onset of early changes of retrolental fibroplasia, it is clear that any measure undertaken to influence the course of the disease must begin now. It must also be mentioned that at least one instance has been recorded (Owens and Owens) where these changes of tortuosity and angiomatous [numerous blood vessels] appearance of the retina have apparently failed to go on to fibroplastic retrolental membrane stage, and reverted to normal. This admittedly is a very remote possibility, but the fact that it has been observed will make interpretation of the beneficial effect of any therapeutic measure just that uncertain . . . it has been decided to try ACTH [adrenocortocotropic hormone] on the rationale that (1) it is a connective tissue disease, (2) prematures may be ACTH-deficient, and (3) no other agent or therapeutic regime has given any indication of beneficial effect.

ACTH was known to produce heightened activity of the adrenal gland and thereby to inhibit proliferation of blood vessels in connective tissue. Thus, it seemed reasonable to expect that the then-new medication might halt the overgrowth of retinal blood vessels in early RLF. However, the previously untried treatment was started more in desperation than conviction. The blood vessel changes in the eyes improved, and the dose was lowered; the changes became worse and the dose was raised. There was improvement, the eyes returned almost to normal, and ACTH was stopped. The infant gained weight, and she was sent home!

Soon after this dramatic experience, 31 infants with early changes of RLF were treated with ACTH at Babies Hospital. Of the 31 infants, 25 left the hospital with normal eyes, 2 became totally blind, 2 lost all vision in one eye, and 2 had useful vision with only minor retinal scars in one or both eyes. Permission for this innovative approach was obtained from the parents in the same informal manner which had been used when another "miracle drug," penicillin, was used to treat life-threatening infections. Each set of parents was told that we had reason to hope that the untried treatment would be effective, but that we were stepping into the unknown. A written document describing the details of study was not drawn up; this was years before the concepts of signed informed consent and review by a Human Investigation Committee were formalized.

Our results of treatment were especially impressive when compared with 7 infants with early RLF at Lincoln Hospital in New York City who did not receive ACTH, 6 of whom had become totally blind. ACTH *seemed* to be the cure for the disease! However, we were puzzled about 2 infants, one at Lincoln Hospital and the other an infant who had been followed by Doctor Blodi; in both, early changes subsided without any treatment and they were left with normal eyes. Our exciting results obviously could not satisfy the simplest rules of evidence. The experience in two different nurseries could not be compared fairly, since it was known that RLF incidence varied widely from hospital to hospital. There was no way to avoid the issue that only a randomized concurrently controlled trial *within each hospital* could definitely settle the ACTH question.

After considerable discussion and soul searching, two formal controlled trials were begun, one at Babies Hospital and the second at Lincoln Hospital. It took only a few months to accumulate the required experience in the premature nurseries of both institutions; a total of 15 infants with early RLF were treated with ACTH and 18 infants observed without treatment. Allotment was decided by drawing from a box containing an equal number of blue and white marbles. Our uncertainty concerning the effectiveness of ACTH was not hidden from the parents, but none were asked to assume our agonizing burden to allow chance to decide on treatment versus nontreatment. Approximately a third of the infants who received ACTH became blind (in one or both eyes) but only one-fifth of the controls went on to blindness. Furthermore, there were more deaths in the ACTH-treated group. When the entire two-year experience of both hospitals was examined, the frequency of cicatricial (scarring) RLF was not startlingly different, but the mortality and morbidity rates were quite disparate; the *untreated* group had fared better.

Two years later, Doctor Owens reported his observations that three-fourths of the infants with early vascular changes of RLF showed *spontaneous* regression to normal. This was exactly our experience in New York during the ACTH-treatment episode.

Following this disheartening experience, a formal experiment was undertaken to test the possibility that premature exposure to light was the cause. Once more the results were negative (see chapter notes).

By mid-1952, after ten years of frustrating activity and false leads, most physicians who were immersed in the study of the RLF epidemic were understandably skeptical of all new claims of cause and cure.

4

The Oxygen Hypothesis

On July 14, 1951, the Medical Journal of Australia printed an article by Kate Campbell of Melbourne, in which she noted

> . . . I heard from colleagues returning from overseas, the suggestion that oxygen might be responsible for producing retrolental fibroplasia. The idea arose apparently from a comparison of the treatment of premature infants in America, where retrolental fibroplasia is a problem and where oxygen was used freely, with the treatment in England, where retrolental fibroplasia is seen rarely, and whole oxygen was used sparingly.

Although Campbell did not identify the source of the suggestion "from overseas," it developed that her informants had visited Birmingham, England, where the recent appearance of RLF was being pondered by V. Mary Crosse and Philip Jameson Evans. In private, Doctor Crosse noted that liberal use of oxygen in England started after the institution of the National Health Service, because government funds now made it possible for hospitals to afford modern incubators and the use of the expensive gas for medical purposes.

As Kinsey and Zacharias had done earlier in Boston (p 19), Crosse and Evans traced the history and course of RLF in England beginning in 1946 and concluded that the occurrence of the disease followed a period of free use of oxygen "on the State," and subsided again with its restriction (Table 4-1). This experience suggested a general political evil to Doctor Evans:

25

. . .as in domestic and national policies, a prolonged subsidy paralyzes the ability to struggle which would otherwise have had the opportunity to develop, and that the disease [RLF] has in fact been artificially induced by a well intentioned, but misguided, change in the management of such cases. That a return to a less indulgent care of the premature infant prevents the disease should be appreciated as soon as possible, and cannot be too quickly undertaken.

Table 4-1
RLF in Birmingham

Period	Number of Infants	Number with RLF
High oxygen[a] (1944– 50)	13	3
Limited oxygen[b] (1951)	6	0

[a]"Free" administration of oxygen (concentration not estimated).

[b]Shortest possible exposure to oxygen, just enough oxygen to prevent cyanosis; graduated return to normal air as soon as possible.

The rise in frequency of RLF coincident with change in oxygen practice in certain hospitals in Melbourne, Australia was reported by Campbell (Table 4-2) and by Ryan, who noted

. . . no case of retrolental fibroplasia had occurred at the Women's Hospital [Melbourne] prior to the introduction of a most efficient oxygen cot. With this apparatus it was the practice of the nursing staff to give oxygen liberally to all babies, even when apparently not requiring it.

On the other hand, Houlton reported that although a rise in RLF did correlate with the use of higher concentrations of oxygen in Oxford, new cases continued to occur even after a reduction in the level of oxygen use.

Thaddeus Szewczyk, an ophthalmologist in East St. Louis, Illinois, postulated that RLF was due to unrecognized oxygen-lack at a time in development when oxygen requirement of the retina was particularly high. He criticized the clinical practice of exposing premature infants to high concentrations of oxygen and subsequent rapid withdrawal in the change from incubator to room air, before acclimation could take place. Szewczyk advised that oxygen be administered to premature infants in minimal amounts and a slow withdrawal from enriched environments. He reported that early changes of RLF appeared when 7 premature infants were moved abruptly from incubators (50-percent oxygen) to bassinettes in room air (21-percent oxygen). Moreover, the changes in the eyes regressed rapidly when the infants were returned to oxygen-rich (60-percent) incubators. In a later trial, blood vessel dilation, new vessel formation and hemorrhages in the retina appeared in 19 premature infants removed rapidly from incubators; when

Table 4-2
RLF in Melbourne

Year	High Oxygen[a] (Institution I)		Moderate Oxygen[b] (Institutions II and III)	
	Number of Infants	*Number With RLF*	*Number of Infants*	*Number With RLF*
1948	36	6	11	2
1949	32	10	23	1
1950	55	7	24	1
Total	123	23	58	4
RLF %	19		7	

[a]In "Institution I" oxygen was piped into the ward and was given in an oxygen cot, in which the percentage of oxygen was 40–60 percent. Oxygen was given prophylactically as well as during periods of cyanosis.

[b]In "Institutions II and III" most, but not all, premature infants were nursed in an electrically heated cot; oxygen was administered by intranasal catheter or funnel, sometimes by tent or cot.

they were returned to high oxygen all improved within 24 hours and their eyes became normal after four days.

However, not all the evidence pointed toward excessive use of oxygen as a cause of RLF. In New Orleans, at a large premature infant center in Charity Hospital, Exline and Harrington examined or traced the outcome in 96 of 131 ex-premature children with very low birthweights (under 1.5 kg = under 3 lb 5 oz) born during a two-year period ending December, 1948. All these children received oxygen at an *estimated* concentration of 50 percent for four or more weeks after birth; none had RLF.

At the Clinique de Puériculture in Paris, two groups of premature infants were compared; in those who received continuous high concentrations of oxygen, the final results (scarring RLF) were no worse than among others raised with a minimum of oxygen (Table 4-3).

While confusion reigned because of the conflicting indications of the role of oxygen from these and other observational studies, a pioneering experimental* clinical trial was undertaken at the Gallinger Municipal Hospital in Washington, D.C. One of the first infants to be placed in a closed incubator in this nursery developed RLF. Leroy Hoeck, the director of the nursery, recalled that the oxygen was delivered through a funnel

*"Experiment is fundamentally induced observation . . . to reason experimentally we must have an idea and afterwards induce or produce facts, i.e., observations to control our preconceived idea."—*Claude Bernard*

Table 4-3
Experience with Oxygen in Paris (1948–1952)

Oxygen Group	Number of Infants	Vascular Changes		Cicatricial RLF	
		No.	Percent	No.	Percent
Highly oxygenated group[a]	344	20	6	21	6
Sparely oxygenated group[b]	135	30	22	11	8

[a]Continuous oxygen (60 percent) never less than 21 days, occasionally 6–8 weeks.

[b]Minimum oxygen (50 percent), discontinuous, given only if indicated for respiratory difficulty or cyanosis; stopped by eighth day at the latest.

strapped to the baby's face. He remarked to Arnall Patz, then a young ophthalmology resident, "All that oxygen might be doing something." Patz recalls that he ". . . explained to Hoeck how unlikely extra oxygen was a factor because the disease seemed to be a response of the type that is associated with anoxia [that is] proliferation of vessels; if indeed, oxygen was related at all." Patz dropped the matter for a while until he came across an article by Stadie describing toxic effects of oxygen on cells, where mention was made of the questionable change in adult retinal vessels upon inhalation of oxygen. In late 1949, toward the end of his hospital residency training, Patz designed a controlled clinical trial and some animal tests, both to explore the idea that excess oxygen might be a factor in causing RLF. With Hoeck, he applied for a research grant of $4000 from the then very small National Institutes of Health for a nursery trial to compare the outcome in infants weighing less than 1.6 kg (under 3½ lb) at birth assigned in alternate order to incubators with either routine oxygen or low oxygen. Oxygen concentration in the incubators was to be monitored by measurement with an electronic analyzer. The grant application was criticized by reviewers as being weak in scientific merit and with extreme concern by the pediatric referees that ". . . these guys are going to kill a lot of babies by anoxia to test a wild idea." Patz and Hoeck satisfied the objections of the referees by stating, "to avoid having deaths from lack of oxygen, every baby in the low oxygen group would be maintained at a healthy pink color." The $4000 was granted.

The nursery trial proved to be difficult for the investigators. Patz found that "The nurses were convinced that we were going to kill the babies in the low oxygen group, and indeed, at night some of the older nurses would turn the oxygen on for a baby who was not receiving oxygen, then turn it off when they would go off duty in the morning." Seventy-six infants were enrolled during the first year of the proposed three-year controlled study; but 11 were dropped from consideration because of technical complications or failure to return for follow-up. The results of the first year's experience were published in 1952; the outcome damned continuous high oxygen (Table 4-4).

Table 4-4
Gallinger Municipal Hospital Controlled Trial of
Oxygen (1952)

Oxygen Administration	Number of Infants	Minor RLF[a]	Severe RLF[b]
High[c]	28	10	7
Low[d]	37	6	0

[a]Blood vessel dilation, tortuosity of retinal vessels, retinal edema, retinal hemorrhages, vitreous clouding.

[b]Detachment of the retina, new vessel formation, retinal hemorrhages, and complete retinal membrane behind the lens in some infants.

[c]65–70 percent oxygen for 4–7 weeks.

[d]Under 40 percent oxygen for 24 hours up to 2 weeks, depending on infant clinical condition, especially cyanosis.

The debates about the role of oxygen were mounting at the end of 1952, and the results of the first controlled trial did not do away with uncertainties in the minds of many observers who were wary after ten years of false leads. Because of the number of infants in the Gallinger Hospital study, concern about the overriding matter of safety of oxygen restriction had not been answered to the satisfaction of many skeptics. Indeed, the survival statistics of the trial were not provided in the report. The bias introduced by alternate case assignment could not be evaluated, and the investigators themselves had a number of unanswered questions about their first experience with a clinical trial. They concluded their report by noting the following:

The data cited here [and the anecdotal reports of others] suggest strongly that high oxygen is a factor in the pathogenesis of retrolental fibroplasia. However, in view of the bizarre manner in which the incidence of the disease fluctuates, additional rigidly controlled observations are necessary to establish this concept.

5

The Eye and Oxygen

In the early 1950s there was a vague feeling that the key to solving the mystery of RLF might lie in improved understanding of the unusual way in which the retinal layer of the eye receives its blood supply during fetal development. Ida Mann, in 1928, described the embryonic development of the human eye and developed the concept that the retinal vessels originate by budding from the base of the fetal blood vessel of the eye (hyaloid artery; see chapter notes). Twenty years later, I. C. Michaelson made observations concerning the fine details of development of the blood vessels and capillaries of the retinal layer. He used a technique which consisted of injecting India ink into the arterial system to fill and blacken the smallest vessels of the fetal eye, removing the globe for dissection, then teasing out the retinal layer to make a flat preparation which he mounted on a glass slide. This allowed him to map the extent of development of patent vessels at different stages of fetal development in a number of species from eels to man.

According to the view established by these observations (see chapter notes for later views), the human retina has no blood supply of its own until the third month of fetal life. This was interpreted to indicate that retinal tissue receives adequate amounts of oxygen and nutrient from the vessels of the choroid layer of the eye which lies just beneath the retina. Michaelson suggested that as the retina develops and becomes thicker at the third to fourth month of gestation, the nutritional needs can no longer be met by the nearby choroid. At the fourth month, a small swelling was seen on the trunk of the hyaloid artery as it passes into the eyeball, at the point where the optic nerve joins the globe. This was considered to be the site of origin of the newly emerging retinal arteries, which appeared to grow outward, reaching the edge of the retina relatively late in the development of the eye.

Michaelson suggested that retinal capillaries sprout from the new vessels which have grown out from the region of the optic nerve. He pointed out that when the veins and arteries are close to one another, capillary growth appears to take place from the side of the vein away from the artery (Fig. 5-1). A capillary network of varying density is seen in the space between the arteries and veins, becoming more abundant as the veins are approached. There is a zone which is free of capillaries around the arteries. Michaelson concluded

. . . there is present in the developing retina a factor which affects the budding of new vessels . . . it is present in a gradient of concentration such that it differs in arterial and venous neighborhoods . . .

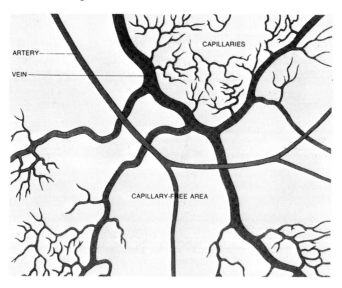

Fig. 5-1.   Appearance of the injected retina of a human fetus, from Michaelson's studies. He considered that capillary growth occurred from the veins forming a capillary-free space around the arteries. Note that the small veins which cross the artery do not branch into capillaries until they have passed the arterial vessel by a certain distance. (Michaelson's concept has been modified by later findings; see chapter notes.)

F. W. Campbell, intrigued by these observations, set out to define Michaelson's "factor." He demonstrated that the capillary-free zones around the arteries in newborn rats (development of the retinal vessel system is similar to that in man) were significantly narrower when the animals were placed in a low-oxygen chamber than in control rats of the same age left in room air. Campbell postulated that an oxygen debt in the developing retina, which can no longer be met by the underlying choroidal vessels, serves as the stimulus for the normal fetal outgrowth of the new system of vessels from the region of the optic nerve. According to this hypothesis, the new blood channels form in response to the growing oxygen needs of the maturing retina.

The relevance of these provocative ideas to RLF went virtually unnoticed for several years. The effects of exposure to low (subatmospheric) oxygen on the immature eye of mice, and the effects of intermittent high oxygen on newborn mice, were reported in 1952. However, abnormal changes in the eye found in these studies were not generally accepted as those of typical human RLF. Young kittens given excessive amounts of salt and water developed swelling of the retinal layer of the eye, but, again, the microscopic appearance of the eyes was not the same as that seen in RLF.

As the nursery controversy concerning the role of oxygen in RLF raged on in 1953, Norman Ashton, a pathologist at the Institute of Ophthalmology, University of London, became interested in the puzzle. He came to the problem with knowledge that the newborn kitten had incomplete blood vessel formation in the retina, roughly comparable to the human premature infant at about 7 months of gestation, and he was armed with the elegant India ink injection technique for retinal study. He borrowed a bacteriology incubator from a pediatrician who had been planning to do some oxygen studies of RLF and converted it to a gas chamber to administer high concentrations of oxygen. With his co-workers, Basil Ward and Geoffrey Serpell, Ashton put a mother cat and three kittens in the chamber and measured the oxygen concentration in the device at half-hour intervals day and night. The first experiment showed that after four days in continuous high oxygen (60–70 percent concentration), the outgrowing retinal vessels were completely withered (Fig. 5-2). The London team went on to demonstrate that constriction of immature vessels was the primary effect of high oxygen. If maintained for a long enough period, obliteration of the entire developing blood vessel network of the retina took place. Regrowth of blood vessels after return to air took place in a wild disorganized fashion with budding of new capillaries into the vitreous portion of the eye in front

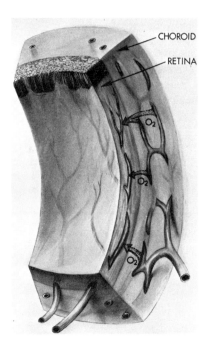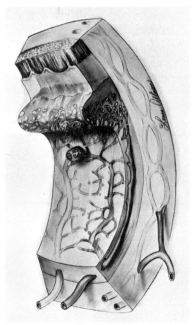

CHOROID

RETINA

Fig. 5-2.   Effect of oxygen in RLF. Left: Initially the retinal vessels are constricted, then obliterated, and peripheral outgrowth is suppressed. Arrows indicate increased diffusion from high oxygen tension in the neighboring choroidal blood vessels, which are not appreciably constricted. Right: Later, the withered blood vessels of the retina regrow in a disorganized fashion; proliferating capillaries erupt through the retinal surface into the vitreous humor. Only the incompletely developed retina is susceptible to this effect of hyperoxia. Once blood vessel development is complete, supplemental oxygen causes a decrease in the caliber of the mature retinal vessels, but pronounced vasoconstriction and obliteration do not take place (see chapter notes, Fig. 9-1, and notes for Chapter 9).

of the retina (Fig. 5-2). This was consistent with the early blood vessel changes in RLF noted in the human by Reese and Blodi in 1951 and amply confirmed by others.

Ashton regarded RLF as no more than a "violent activation" of the normal process of retinal vessel development, precipitated by an exaggerated lack of oxygen in the deep retinal layers, as described earlier by Campbell. Ironically and paradoxically, it was exposure to high oxygen concentration, with resultant obliteration of developing retinal blood vessels, which appeared to cause the ultimate oxygen deficiency in the deep retinal layer of the eye. These results seemed bizarre: breathing high concentrations of oxygen appeared to render one tissue of the body oxygen-impoverished! On the other hand, the findings also provided a basis for some reconciliation with the views of those who considered overall oxygen-lack to be the cause of RLF. Although Ashton's experiments indicated that low oxygen, consistent with the survival of his animals, usually was not sufficient to give rise to proliferation of retinal blood vessels, he suggested the possiblity that *severe* oxygen-lack might, on occasion, produce the disease directly.

In 1953, Patz and his co-workers conducted extensive studies of high oxygen exposure in several species of newborn animals, beginning with opossum and rats and later with mice, kittens, and puppies, with the same results as those reported by Ashton. Although these elegant animal studies were impressive, there was one substantial problem in extending the findings to human RLF; this was voiced by Ashton:

> The findings exactly parallel the early stages of the human disease. The difference in subsequent course is dependent upon the development of retinal detachment which did not occur in the kitten experiments.

In other words, the blood vessel changes of RLF in newborn kittens and other experimental animals did not go on to scarring (cicatricial) RLF. The experimental animals did not become blind!

By the beginning of 1953, the next step seemed clear to me and to many of my peers who were responsible for the day-to-day care of premature infants. We were worried about the harmful consequences of oxygen restriction and felt that further study in *babies* was the only way to resolve the substantial doubt concerning the exact role of oxygen in human RLF.

6

The National Cooperative Study

By the year 1953, approximately 10,000 children had been blinded by RLF, 7000 of whom were born in the United States. Government agencies and private organizations were gearing up for the greatly increased need for special facilities. At the same time, they (notably the National Society for the Prevention of Blindness) clamored for action to halt the epidemic. The most promising clue to the solution of the problem lay with the evidence against the use of supplemental oxygen.

At the 1952 meeting of the American Academy of Ophthalmology and Otolaryngology the idea was conceived of organizing a national cooperative study. Spurred by V. Everett Kinsey, a research biochemist then at the Kresge Eye Institute in Detroit, and Franklin M. Foote, then Director of the National Society for the Prevention of Blindness, a large meeting was convened in Bethesda, Maryland, early in 1953 under the auspices of the National Institute of Neurological Diseases and Blindness of the U.S. Public Health Service. Also in attendance were most of the American pediatricians and ophthalmologists who had been studying the RLF epidemic.

It soon became clear that there were two camps. The majority felt that a formal controlled trial must be carried out immediately to answer the outstanding questions concerning oxygen treatment. A minority felt that there was sufficient evidence to indict oxygen therapy as the cause of RLF, and argued that the proposal for a new nursery study was not justified, and even immoral. The dissidents cited the results of the only properly controlled trial (p 27). However, the majority were impressed that the persons who conducted the Gallinger Hospital trial and knew its defects were solidly on the side of the cooperative study. One splinter group felt that *limiting* oxygen would require, infants to undertake an unjustified risk of death and brain damage. After much debate, most of it heated, it was agreed that a joint effort should be undertaken to determine whether the frequency of occurrence of RLF is dependent upon the amount of oxygen used in the management of premature infants. An eight-man subcommittee (Appendix B) was appointed to draw up specific plans for the cooperative study.

The planners met in Atlantic City in spring 1953 and debated the dilemma, i.e., whether the administration of substantially lesser amounts of oxygen might increase mortality, or whether continued use of the customary amounts might result in an unnecessarily high frequency of RLF. In the end, a strategy was chosen with the intention of minimizing both risks:

> [Only] one-twelfth of the total number of infants expected to be in the study was to be assigned to the . . . routine [unrestricted] oxygen group. In this way, should oxygen indeed prove to be positively associated with retrolental fibroplasia, the number of infants in the participating hospitals who would receive routine [unrestricted] oxygen during the . . . [study period] would be substantially less than normal. To obtain an answer to the questionable role of oxygen as soon as possible whilst not materially sacrificing [concurrent]temporal controls, one infant was to be assigned to the routine, [unrestricted] oxygen group for every two babies assigned to curtailed oxygen group during the first three months of the study. If at the end of the [first] three-month period there was *no difference in mortality* [italics added], all babies were to be assigned to the curtailed group until such time as the incidence of retrolental fibroplasia in the two groups could be evaluated.

(For further details of the study design see chapter notes.)

Eighteen hospitals (Appendix C) agreed to abide by a uniform protocol which was drawn up by the Coordinating Committee for the treatment of infants. The study began on July 1, 1953, and continued until June 30, 1954. Infants who weighed 1.5 kg or less ($\leq$ 3 lb 5 oz) and who survived 48 hours were enrolled in the study. The Coordination Center at Kresge Eye Institute, Detroit, was notified by telegram of the entry of each infant and assignment to a treatment category was made by return telegram. Until 68 infants were assigned to the "routine oxygen" (unrestricted) group, assignment was made in separate sets of 3 infants for each hospital—1 infant was allotted to the routine oxygen group for every 2 infants assigned to the "curtailed-oxygen" treatment category, the order of assignment randomized within each set of 3.

Mortality rates in the two oxygen-treatment groups were monitored week by week. Three months after the trial began, there appeared to be no systematic difference in survival between infants in the curtailed-oxygen group and the 68 infants who had been enrolled in routine oxygen; according to the prearranged plan all subsequent infants received curtailed-oxygen and enrollment continued for nine more motnhs. A total of 786 premature infants were admitted to the Cooperative Study; 166 died prior to 40 days, and the eyes of 34 were not examined adequately (i.e., for a minimum follow-up of 2½ months after birth); this left 586 infants in whom the relationship between oxygen treatment and RLF could be analyzed.

As the Cooperative Study proceeded there was understandable impatience for information among all concerned in the trial and in the medical community at large. But, in view of the many dashed hopes in the checkered history of the RLF epidemic, all participants in the investigation agreed that no results should be released until the carefully planned trial was completed and all the accumulated data were analyzed; September 1954 was considered to be the earliest date for a responsible report. As a result there was considerable consternation among all concerned when a memorandum was circulated to hospitals with maternity and newborn services in New York City, dated April, 1954; it read (in part)

> Recent studies suggest a possible interrelationship between high concentrations of oxygen and the development of retrolental fibroplasia in premature infants. It has therefore been recommended by the Pediatric Advisory Committee that premature infants receive oxygen only as needed and then in concentrations not to exceed 40 per cent

The bulletin did not identify the "recent studies," but clearly the Cooperative Study was not being cited. The physicians who were participating in the national study were baffled by this turn of events. The minutes of the meeting of the Pediatric Advisory Committee of the New York City Health Department, dated March 18, 1954, shed no light on the source of the information which led to the action of this group.

In May 1954, another document added to the apprehensions of those who were awaiting the results of the national study. A randomized controlled clinical trial was reported which compared the effects of high versus low oxygen therapy among 64 surviving premature infants at Bellevue Hospital. The results clearly indicted high oxygen. However, puzzled skeptics raised questions which were not answered in the publication. For example, the report did not mention the Cooperative Study which was underway, despite the fact that Bellevue Hospital was one of the 18 cooperating hospitals in the national effort. Since the calendar dates of the trial period were not reported, it was unclear whether (1) the Bellevue report included some infants who were also enrolled in the Cooperative Study, in which case the interpretation would be clouded by a number of irreconcilable problems, real and/or theoretical, or (2) the trial reported in May 1954 had been completed before the national study, in which case it was difficult to understand why the Bellevue group joined the 18-hospital national effort. Although it would seem that an explanation would be simple to find, to this day the exact circumstances are unclear.

The safety of oxygen restriction was not established convincingly by the Bellevue controlled trial. Mortality in the low-oxygen group was greater than in the group that received oxygen liberally, but the difference was thought to be explained by chance. The authors concluded from this evidence and from a review of their uncontrolled experience during the previous 10 years that a policy of oxygen restriction did not appear to be harmful. Many observers, noting the small number of infants in the Bellevue study, chose to await the results of the National Cooperative Study before altering the methods of care for premature infants which might increase mortality or brain damage.

In the Bellevue trial, infants in the low oxygen group who required oxygen received it from prepared tanks containing a mixture of 50-percent oxygen and 50-percent nitrogen to prevent accidental administration of higher concentrations of oxygen. The concentration of oxygen measured in incubators when this gas mix was administered averaged 38 percent (standard deviation ± 7.7 percent). Among 28 infants assigned to the low oxygen group, there was no cicatricial (scarring) RLF. These results led the authors to propose giving oxygen only to definitely cyanotic infants, and then at measured concentrations below 40 percent. This ceiling was the same as that advised in the April 1954 recommendation of the New York City Health Department.

Two other reports appeared in 1954 while the national trial was underway, and raised the debates concerning oxygen therapy to new heights of intensity. In the first report, from Philadelphia, the effects of rapid versus slow withdrawal from oxygen were evaluated by a controlled trial. However, each infant who developed progressive RLF was, in the authors' words, ". . . placed back in oxygen at the same concentration from which he had been removed. Because our results with oxygen therapy had been uniformly successful, we did not feel it was fair to withhold treatment in order to obtain control cases . . ." Although the results of this experience condemned excessive use of oxygen (and rapid withdrawal from oxygen in particular), many observers found it very difficult to interpret the results because of the confounding factor introduced by oxygen "treatment" of early RLF.

The second report reviewed the experience at the Colorado General Hospital from 1947 through 1953. Coincident rise and fall of RLF frequency with increase and decrease in use of oxygen was similar to experiences reported by some, but not all, others. The experience was widely quoted even before it was published, principally because the retrospective analysis of mortality led the highly respected authors to the conclusion that oxygen restriction was safe.

The suspense which preceded the first announcement of the Cooperative Study was almost unbearable to those who had waited so long for a definitive answer to their questions. They were not disappointed. On September 19, 1954, at the Fifty-Ninth Annual Session of the American Academy of Ophthalmology and Otolaryngology in New York City, Kinsey presented the preliminary results (Table 6-1), and all doubt concerning the causal role of oxygen in RLF seemed to be dispelled. Mortality among infants allotted to the two contrasting oxygen-therapy groups was declared "not significantly different" (see chapter notes).

Table 6-1

Frequency of RLF in the Cooperative Study, By Multiplicity of Birth and Severity of RLF (July 1, 1953–June 30, 1954)

		Singleton			
		Blood Vessel			
	Number of	Changes of RLF		Scarring RLF	
Oxygen Group	Infants	No.	%	No.	%
Routine oxygen	47	33	70	8	17
Curtailed oxygen	425	133	31	20*	5
		Multiple Birth			
Routine oxygen	6	5	83	4	67
Curtailed oxygen	108	45	42	15*	14

*These little-remembered details of the one-year trial deserve emphasis: Not all of the infants who received "curtailed" oxygen in 1953–54 escaped without RLF. There were 35 instances of scarring (cicatricial) RLF among infants in the "curtailed" group, compared with 12 infants who incurred residual lesions in the "routine oxygen" group.

When the final report of the Cooperative Study was released several unsuspected associations were disclosed; for example,

—scarring (cicatricial) RLF occurred about three times more frequently in twins (and other multiple-birth infants) than in singletons, despite the fact that on the average, the latter received oxygen for longer periods and had a lower gestational age than the multiple-birth infants;

—the frequency of cicatricial RLF was not dependent upon the concentration of oxygen administered, but increased rapidly with increased *duration* of exposure to oxygen, particularly for the first few days of exposure. The risk increased with exposure for periods of up to 2 weeks for multiple birth infants;

—for all practical purposes, there was no concentration of oxygen above that in room air which was not associated with risk of developing RLF;

—the rate of withdrawal from oxygen did not appear to play a primary role in the development of changes leading to RLF.

(See chapter notes for a comparison of these results with those found in animal studies.)

The epidemic of RLF came to a dramatic halt following widespread publicity given to the report of the Cooperative Study. The Great Oxygen Debate all but ceased.

7

Oxygen Treatment Practices in Premature Infant Care

The practice of administering supplemental oxygen to premature infants began many years before the onset of the RLF epidemic. Inadequate oxygen supply to the tissues is one of the most frequent and most ominous complications in prematurely born infants. This grave difficulty was obvious, even to the unaided eye of caretakers in the past, because of the dramatic color change of the skin from a healthy pink to a sickly blue hue, the color of insufficiently oxygenated arterial blood. This symptom, cyanosis, may be caused by a number of lifethreatening disorders of vital organs (especially lungs and heart), but also occurs in association with inexplicable episodes of cessation of breathing in otherwise normal premature infants.

Budin, in 1900, recommended oxygen inhalation for cyanotic episodes in premature infants. In 1917, Ylppö advised that oxygen be introduced into the stomach by tube as a means of resuscitating premature infants and to manage apnea (arrested breathing). The method was used widely in Scandanavia and in England for many years. In 1922, Hess noted a method, described in 1912, of injecting oxygen under the skin for asphyxial (suffocation) attacks in infants, but he rejected this approach. He recommended, instead, that "The oxygen tank should be kept at the side of the infant's bed and either continuous or intermittent showers of oxygen given

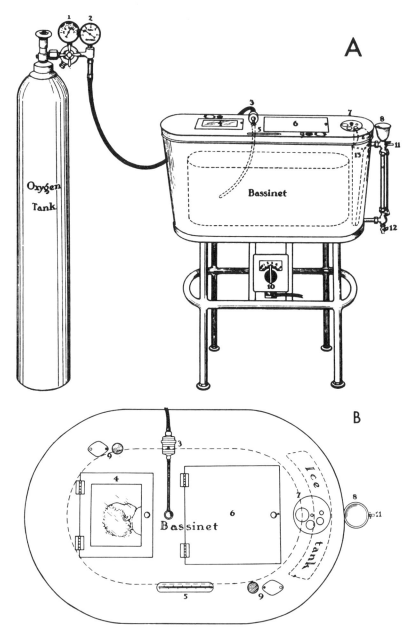

Fig. 7-1. Hess bed equipped with an oxygen therapy unit (A–side and B–top views). 1.—Pressure gauge, 2.—oxygen flow regulator, 3.—flow meter 4.—glass and metal hinged door for feeding purposes, 5.—thermometer window, 6.—metal hinged door for purposes of body care of the infant, 7.—ventilator with small and large exit openings, 8–12.—controls for maintaining temperature in water-jacket of the incubator.

44

in the attempt to ward off cyanotic attacks." In 1923, Bakwin studied cyanotic attacks in premature infants and demonstrated that these could be relieved by oxygen inhalations. He noted that when oxygen was administered early, subsequent cyanotic attacks were fewer in number and more readily amenable to treatment. To reap full benefit from treatment, Bakwin recommended that oxygen be given over a long period of time, preferably in a closed chamber.

Hess described an infant oxygen unit, which was used in the Sarah Morris Premature Infant Station beginning in 1931 (Fig. 7-1), in which 346 of 792 infants admitted to the nursery over a three-year period were placed. The indications for treatment were suffocation after resuscitation of the newborn infant, cyanosis, and various lung infections. Oxygen was administered for more than 24 hours, and occasionally as long as 6 weeks. Concentration of oxygen (predicted from flow meter settings, see chapter notes) was usually "40 percent"; in a few instances this was increased to "50–55 percent." The oxygen policies were credited, in part, for improved survival (Table 7-1).

As noted in Chapter 2, skilled, highly opinionated nurses dominated the scene in hospital nurseries before the 1940s. Physicians played a minor role; they entered the nurseries for brief periods, wrote fairly general orders for care, and trusted the specialized nurses to make detailed minute-by-minute decisions concerning clinical management. In the use of supplemental oxygen as a life-saving measure for premature infants, the opinions of "old hands" carried considerable weight. Nurses' opinions were translated into practice for most of the 70 or so years during which oxygen had been available in hospitals.

Opinion/practice in the matter of oxygen treatment of premature infants can be divided into fairly distinct epochs. In the first period, it was the conventional wisdom that supplemental oxygen improved chances for

Table 7-1

Survival of Premature Infants Before and After Infant
Oxygen Unit, Sarah Morris Premature Infant Station, Chicago

Years	Number of Infants Admitted	Number Which Survived	Survival (%)
Before oxygen unit:			
1922–1926	266	138	52
1927–1929	495	335	68
After oxygen unit:			
1931–1933	792	628	79

survival of infants with "asphyxial attacks." This opinion was led by Madame Louise Recht, the Budin-trained nurse who traveled widely in the United States during the years 1903–1950 (p 15), and Miss Evelyn Lundeen, the dean of American newborn-nursing experts who was Doctor Hess' head nurse for many years. They firmly supported the view that oxygen treatments were life-saving. Their indications for oxygen were cyanosis and other fairly obvious manifestations of lack.

The second period of oxygen opinion/practice began with observations made in Detroit at the Children's Hospital of Michigan in 1942. Attention was directed to (1) subtle indicators of the need for supplemental oxygen, and (2) the effects of high concentration of the gas. The breathing characteristics of 33 *healthy* premature infants were recorded while breathing room air. Of these, 25 breathed in a well-recognized regular–irregular pattern known as "periodic breathing." when 28 of these asymptomatic infants were placed in a 70-percent oxygen atmosphere, 23 shifted to a regular type of breathing (Fig. 7-2). The authors concluded that

> We have no proof that the regular type of respiration which we are accustomed to consider "normal" is "better" for a premature infant than the periodic breathing described. Likewise, we have no convincing evidence that an increased oxygen content of arterial blood is beneficial or necessarily of importance. It is evident, however, that these healthy premature infants breathed in a more normal manner in an oxygen enriched atmosphere.

Also in 1942, Smith and Kaplan reported that the color of the skin in the premature infant was often an unreliable indicator of the state of oxygenation of the blood. Twenty-three premature infants studied between birth and 26 days of life had oxygen saturation levels in blood which were lower than those found in adults or in full-term infants of comparable age; the relatively low levels were not accompanied by a visible blue tinge of the skin. They suggested that the premature infant may be in a state of "subcyanotic anoxia" (oxygen-lack without the tell-tale sign of blue skin color, perhaps as the result of the fact that blood in the capillaries of the skin receives some oxygen directly from the surrounding air by diffusion through the thin epidermis). These observations provided a rationale for the administration of oxygen to asymptomatic premature infants to reduce the risk of brain damage caused by unrecognized oxygen lack.

At the end of World War II, incubators were designed and built to meet the new specifications of physicians for high-oxygen-concentration capability and improved visibility in the incubator to permit direct observation of the breathing characteristics of premature infants. The Isolette,

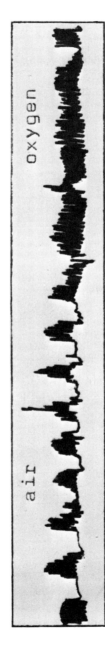

Fig. 7-2. Breathing patterns of a healthy, small premature infant. A "periodic" pattern in room air, "regular" in 70-percent oxygen.

developed by engineers of the newly formed Air-Shields Company, was the predecessor of the new generation of infant incubators (Fig. 7-3). It was adapted from the design of Chapple, which called for a tightly gasketed chamber ventilated with large volumes of air drawn by a circulating fan from out-of-hospital (or filtered nursery) air to assure outflow of air, thus barring the entrance of nursery air through access ports. This design effectively isolated the infant from airborne contamination, but it did create a problem when high concentrations of oxygen were ordered; dilution of the

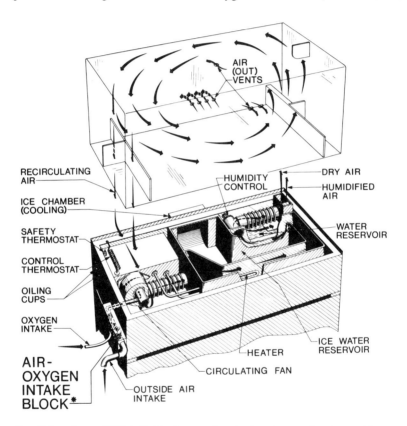

Fig. 7-3. A pre-1954 individually ventilated Chapple-type incubator (blow-up view). Air was drawn into the incubator at the rate of 10 liters per minute to prevent the accumulation of carbon dioxide produced by the infant occupant and to bar the entrance of nursery air when the access ports were opened to care for the infant. The plexiglass hood made the respiratory movements of the naked infant in the incubator highly visible to attendants. *See details of air–oxygen intake block in Fig. 7-4.

administered gas with outside air would require a very large oxygen flow to raise oxygen concentration. A rectangular plenum (Fig. 7-4) was designed to solve this technical problem. When outside air was used alone, it was sucked through a screen filter; the air then proceeded through the blower into the heating chamber of the incubator. A cylinder-shaped space above an oxygen nipple housed a small two-tiered float, weighted and designed so that when oxygen was used the flow of this gas raised the float-valve, gradually restricting the intake of outside air. Under these conditions oxygen concentration rose rapidly and permitted efficient use of the expensive gas.

On the day the results of the Cooperative Study were made known to the Air-Shields Company, the president sent a memorandum to every hospital in the world which used the Isolette incubator; it read, in part,

Recommendation—removal of the small float in the air–oxygen intake assembly.

In February 1955, the New York State Health Department mailed an information memorandum on RLF to all health officers, chiefs of medical staffs and hospital administrators in the state (excluding New York City). The bulletin called attention to published articles and editorials implicating oxygen treatment and announced a forthcoming publication which would discuss the control of oxygen therapy to premature infants. The Health Department document noted that "Blindness due to retrolental fibroplasia appears to be entirely preventable . . . If oxygen is administered to prema-

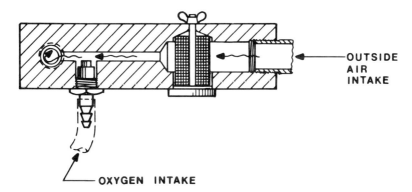

Fig. 7-4.   Air–oxygen intake assembly of the pre-1954 model Isolette incubator. A two-tiered float valve was raised by the flow of oxygen to restrict the flow of diluting outside air into the incubator.

ture infants (when clinically indicated rather than routinely), concentrations should be kept below 40%." The promised article appeared in May 1955; in it, Doctor Lanman of Bellevue Hospital advised that "Oxygen therapy should be given only to infants with clinical signs of respiratory distress and then for as short a time as possible. Concentration should never exceed 40 percent oxygen." Soon similar advice was given in bulletins, memoranda, and regulations of Health Departments in states and cities throughout the country.

Apart from reasonable doubt about such black-and-white precision on strictly biologic grounds, these statements and recommendations were surprising in view of evidence which had already been made available in the Cooperative Study. As described (p 41) it had been shown that (1) RLF *did* occur in infants assigned to curtailed oxygen (Table 6-1), and (2) there was no threshold concentration of oxygen which delineated the risk of developing RLF. A later paper from Bellevue, entitled "The Possibility of Total Elimination of Retrolental Fibroplasia by Oxygen Restriction," again advised that oxygen concentrations only under 40 percent be used. Then Kinsey wrote a letter to the editor objecting to the emphasis which was being placed on the concentration of oxygen:

I have learned that a number of pediatricians have gained the impression that there is appreciably less risk of developing RLF if oxygen is administered at less than 40% concentration . . . In view of the paucity of evidence that there is any critical concentration below which RLF is markedly reduced in incidence, I believe that merely restricting the concentration of oxygen without stringently reducing the duration in oxygen, may result in unnecessary cases of RLF. Certainly the emphasis should be placed on restricting duration in oxygen to an absolute minimum consistent with clinical indications of anoxia irrespective of the concentration of oxygen administered.

Harry Gordon was also prompted to comment on the issue of oxygen restriction. He pointed out that the conclusions of the Cooperative Study concerning the relation of oxygen restriction to the survival rate of premature infants presented a problem:

In the [Cooperative Study] report, it is pointed out that infants were admitted to the study only if they survived 48 hours, and that the *mortality figures refer to infants who had already survived the first 2 days of life* [italics added] . . . Since the risk of dying from anoxia [oxygen lack] is greatest for premature infants during the first 48 hours, it is obvious that a conclusion such as the one stated [limitation is without an effect on survival] may be misleading.

These warnings by Kinsey and by Gordon went largely unheeded. An epoch of oxygen opinion/practice, which may be called the "under-40%-era," was ushered in at the end of 1954. Concentrations of oxygen administered to premature infants were carefully monitored by serial measurements in the incubators and so long as the concentration remained below 40 percent, many felt secure that the infant was safely and properly protected from the risk of RLF.

8

The Consequences of Oxygen Restriction

Interest in RLF quickly waned after 1955. Except for the engrossment of tort lawyers, very little attention was paid to the condition (Fig. 8-1). Governmental plans for developing expanded facilities for blind children were quietly shelved and there was general agreement that RLF could be chalked up in the "solved" column.

As noted, the under-40%-only policy of oxygen treatment was adopted widely; indeed, it was reinforced by the knowledge that malpractice suits for RLF were burgeoning. Within a short time, however, it became evident that total elimination of RLF could not be realized; some cases continued to occur after 1954–1955. As might have been predicted from the pre-1940 history of the disorder, typical and fully documented instances of RLF occurred in some premature infants who had never received supplemental oxygen. Although this occurred rarely and was first doubted by many, the weight of evidence was finally convincing and the possibility was accepted that 21-percent oxygen in ordinary room air can "produce" RLF. When RLF occurred in infants who were exposed to oxygen very briefly (e.g. only during resuscitation at birth), it created endless arguments about cause and effect. Most of the debates were occurring in front of juries hearing numerous malpractice suits tried in the years after 1954.

The first sign of a backlash effect from the new restrictive practice of

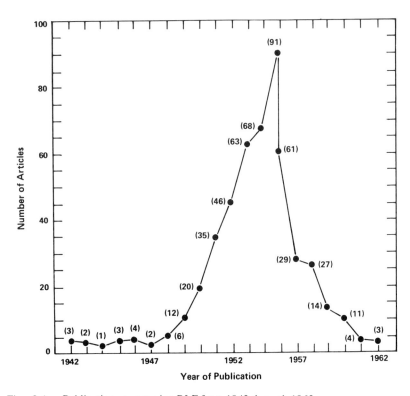

Fig. 8-1.   Publications concerning RLF from 1942 through 1962.

oxygen treatment appeared more than 5 years after announcement of the results of the Cooperative Study. Mary Ellen Avery and Ella H. Oppenheimer reviewed autopsies at Johns Hopkins Hospital noting the mortality and frequency of occurrence of the commonest life-threatening complication in premature infants: hyaline membrane disease. (Respiratory distress syndrome is the label applied to a serious breathing problem caused by inadequate stabilizing substance - surfactant - in the lung. In those infants with respiratory distress who die, most have a transparent, membrane-like deposit in the lung which gives the condition its pathologic name: hyaline membrane disease.) The Baltimore investigators reasoned that if the lung condition was the result of incomplete development and unrelated to factors that operate after birth, frequency should be essentially the same from one period of time to the next. Further, they postulated that since there was no definitive treatment, the mortality rate associated with hyaline membrane disease should remain practically constant. However, when they examined the experience of two 5-year periods, they found a definite change; frequency of hyaline membrane disease and mortality were both higher during the years of oxygen sparing (Table 8-1). The authors wisely refrained from applying statistical tests to the retrospective review and cautiously concluded the following:

> The increase in the number of deaths from hyaline membrane disease in the period of restricted oxygen use suggests that some infants with respiratory distress may need more oxygen than they have been receiving.

They warned that the observations pertained only to deaths from hyaline membrane disease (but this is the most frequent single cause of death after premature birth). In retrospect, it is curious that the report made no mention of the Gordon letter, which had been published three years earlier and had called attention to the problem of interpreting the conclusions of the Cooperative Study concerning the safety of oxygen restriction (p 50). Even more surprising, the understated, but nonetheless disturbing, observations from Johns Hopkins Hospital evoked relatively little response in neonatal circles. No other publicized review of the association between oxygen policy change and mortality appeared for 14 years (p 62).

In 1962 Alison D. McDonald reported the results of the follow-up examinations of 1081 English ex-premature children at ages 6 to 8 years.

Table 8-1

Mortality and Occurrence of Hyaline Membrane Disease in
Two 5-Year Periods (Johns Hopkins Hospital
Premature Nursery)

Years	Number of Births[a]	Deaths[b] No.	%	Hyaline Membrane Disease[c] No.	As % of Births	As % of Autopsies
1944–1948[d]	1152	95	8	17	2	24
1954–1958[e]	1492	186	13	56	4	39

[a]Birthweight 1.0–2.5 kg (2 lb 4 oz–5 lb 8 oz).

[b]From 30 min to 6 days of age.

[c]Hyaline membrane disease was determined by the microscopic appearance of lungs. All slides were reviewed, retrospectively, by the same pathologist.

[d]Oxygen concentration was not measured during this period but almost all premature infants received oxygen at a rate sufficient to produce a concentration of 60–80%. There was a high frequency of RLF during this period.

[e]Because the role of oxygen in RLF was "defined," pediatricians were reluctant to raise the oxygen concentration in incubators to more than 40 percent.

These children who had weighed 1.8 kg (4 lb) or less at birth had been studied earlier in a nationwide investigation of RLF by the Medical Research Council. McDonald sought to discover associations between perinatal events and the occurrence of spastic diplegia, known to occur more often following premature birth than after term delivery. A relatively high rate of diplegia, and low rates of other types of cerebral palsy, were found in this group of ex-premature children. No associations were observed between diplegia and various complications of pregnancy and delivery (e.g., neither asphyxia during delivery nor resuscitation). However, there was a correlation between spastic diplegia and a history of postnatal breathing difficulties associated with cyanotic spells and respiratory distress (as indicated by retractions of the chest wall and grunting respiration). There was also a relationship between the neurologic outcome and the duration of oxygen therapy with an opposing trend as to the status of the eyes, i.e., spastic diplegia frequency fell and RLF rose as the duration of oxygen treatment increased (Fig. 8-2). Doctor McDonald concluded that

> There was some indication that prolonged oxygen therapy prevented diplegia in very immature infants with cyanotic attacks. It is suggested that this treatment may be of value if retrolental fibroplasia can be avoided.

A similar follow-up of children who had been enrolled in the American Cooperative Study was planned but never carried out (p 63).

In the early 1960s there was increasing uneasiness with the blanket policy of oxygen restriction for all premature infants. Although the cited reviews played a part in raising these doubts, the tide of opinion/practice was turned by the flood of new information which became available following the technical development making it possible to measure the partial pressure of oxygen in small samples of arterial blood (see chapter notes).

From the outset, when high oxygen had been accepted as the cause of RLF, it seemed unreasonable that oxygen surrounding the infant would be more critical than the oxygen in the blood vessels. When arterial blood oxygen tension in premature infants with respiratory distress syndrome (p 60) was correlated with oxygen in inspired air, it was evident that many of these babies were inadequately oxygenated while breathing 40-percent oxygen (see chapter notes for further details). Studies at Oxford in 1962 demonstrated that most infants with severe respiratory difficulty required very high concentrations of oxygen in inspired air to raise the oxygen level of aortic blood. Further studies suggested that prompt resuscitation and exposure to high concentrations of oxygen (80–90 percent) in premature infants with asphyxia of the newborn (due to inadequate exchange of

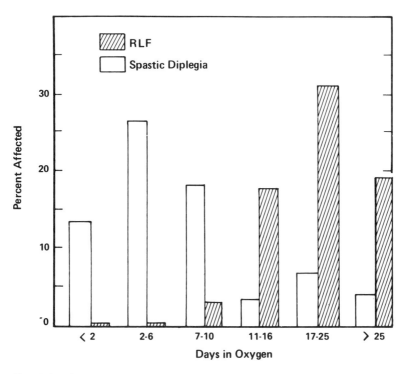

Fig. 8-2. Spastic diplegia and RLF according to median duration of oxygen treatment. Among 194 children born before 31 weeks gestation who had increasing duration of oxygen therapy, spastic diplegia occurred less frequently, but RLF turned up more frequently. There was no association between spastic diplegia and duration of oxygen administration in children born after longer periods of gestation.

oxygen and carbon dioxide between the fetus and the mother across the placenta before delivery, or failure of the newborn infant to breathe promptly after birth) might forestall the development of the respiratory distress syndrome. These observations provided the rationale for a liberalization in the mid-1960s of the restrictive policy of oxygen therapy, but there was serious concern that premature infants might be subjected to an increased risk of RLF.

In 1967 the National Society for the Prevention of Blindness convened a meeting of 28 American and Canadian pediatricians, ophthalmologists and biophysicists to consider the problems posed by the new shift in oxygen opinion/practice. The discussion centered on the need for the following:

1. Criteria for supplemental oxygen administration;
2. Accumulating evidence on the association of clinical signs, arterial oxygen measurements, appearance of retina through the ophthalmo-scope, and status of brain function in oxygen-treated infants;
3. Improvement of devices for monitoring oxygen concentration in the air breathed by newborn infants;
4. Caution in administering supplemental oxygen when appropriate ob-servations cannot be made;
5. Basic research in factors which control blood vessel function.

Humbled by the fact that only anecdotal clinical evidence was available, the participants wisely refrained from making definite recommendations concerning the treatment of premature infants. However they agreed, tacitly, that a definite change in opinion/practice had once more taken place.

9

The Determinative Era of Oxygen Treatment

The most recent epoch of opinion/practice concerning oxygen therapy began hesitantly in the 1960s. It slowly became apparent that the old fears of experienced nurses in the early 1950s had not been entirely groundless. The use of oxygen in the treatment of premature infants with obvious signs of oxygen deficiency posed a classic Scylla-and-Charybdis-like dilemma for physicians. Liberal administration was thought to increase the risk of RLF, whereas restricted use was expected to increase mortality and the likelihood of brain damage in survivors. Repeated determinations of the state of oxygenation of each sick infant seemed the obvious approach to guide treatment and avoid impalement on this two horned dilemma in the nursery.

The monitoring of treatment by direct ophthalmoscopy to detect oxygen-induced narrowing of retinal arteries proved to be impractical at a time when information was needed most. Examination of desperately ill infants in the first hours and days of life was difficult for the examiner and dangerously exhausting for the patients. Moreover, visualization of the retina was often blurred by vitreal haze.

The Nuffield Neonatal Research Unit at the Hammersmith Hospital in London proposed a plan, the pure oxygen breathing test (Table 9-1), which gained fairly wide acceptance. This scheme formalized a trend already underway, a shift of attention from the concentration of oxygen in inspired air to the measurement of oxygen tension in serial samples of arterial blood (usually from the aorta via an umbilical artery catheter). The question of whether there was a threshold arterial condition (elevated oxygen tension over a period of time) for RLF to develop was as difficult to answer as the earlier poser when oxygen was measured in inspired air only. Although it seemed reasonable to attempt to control blood oxygen tension at the levels found in "normal" infants breathing room air (about 60– 100 mm Hg), it would have been surprising if this eliminated RLF completely since, as I have already indicated, there were documented examples of the disorder in infants who had never received supplemental oxygen. Indeed, the Hammersmith group encountered RLF in an infant whose oxygen tension (in serial samples of arterial blood) never measured more than 80 mm Hg. The unanswered question remained, Will the new "determinative" policy be associated with an increased frequency of RLF?

There was no national data-pool in the United States from which the ongoing incidence of RLF could be determined. Blind or visually impaired children in a community were usually not reported to service agencies until they appeared for schooling. Thus, there was an agonizing lag of 5 years or more before a rise in frequency could be detected unless the increase was explosive. In this uneasy atmosphere of doubt and concern, I approached the National Society for the Prevention of Blindness and suggested that a survey be conducted to attempt early detection of any rise in the occurrence of RLF: The year 1967 was chosen as a representative one for the new oxygen practices.

Table 9-1

Breathing Pure Oxygen: A Test To Determine Oxygen
Treatment In Respiratory Distress Syndrome

Arterial Oxygen While Breathing Pure Oxygen[a]	Recommended Change in Oxygen Treatment
< 100[b]	Remain in 90– 100% oxygen[c]
100– 150	Decrease in 10% steps (remeasure)
150– 300	Decrease in 20% steps (remeasure)
> 300	Decrease in 40% steps (remeasure)

[a]Partial pressure of oxygen (in millimeters of mercury) in blood drawn from the aorta through an umbilical artery catheter, after the infant has been breathing pure oxygen by face mask for 15 minutes.

[b]Asymptomatic infants breathing room air have arterial oxygen measurements ranging from about 60 mm Hg at birth to about 100 mm Hg at 54 hours of age.

[c]Administered in a Plexiglass box enclosing the infant's head.

Some 1100 North American hospitals were canvassed by mail with a request for the numbers of infants with RLF born in the survey year. Only 369 of the hospitals responded, and the crude estimate of frequency of occurrence provided no clear answer to the question. The fact that only 33 examples of RLF were uncovered was not reassuring. On the contrary, the results suggested that many infants-at-risk were not being examined in 1967.

Beginning in 1969, five hospitals throughout the United States undertook a forward-seeking, collaborative study to determine the "safe" arterial oxygen tension to reduce the risk of RLF. The goal was not realized. Observations in 719 infants, most of whom were being treated for respiratory distress, indicated that there was no significant difference in average oxygen tension in infants who developed cicatricial RLF and those whose eyes remained normal. In both groups average arterial oxygen values did not exceed the "normal range" (60–100 mm of mercury).

Recent findings have compounded the problem of deciding whether or not the incidence of RLF has been increasing during the late 1960s and 1970s among premature infants (particularly those with moderate or no respiratory symptoms who were exposed to relatively little supplemental oxygen). Improved techniques (retinal photography, indirect ophthalmoscopy, and fluorescein angiography) for examining the retinas of newborn infants have shown that the blood vessel changes of RLF (Fig. 9-1) occur much more often than appreciated in the past. It seems unlikely that the high frequency is explained entirely by latter-day liberal oxygen practices. For example, Baum found many residual changes in the eyes of 52 late-teenagers in Denver, Colorado, who had been born prematurely during the years before and after oxygen restriction. He observed only three persons with normal eyes, 14 had some degree of cicatricial (scarring) RLF, and 35 showed abnormal twists and turns of the retinal arteries (Fig. 9-2).

From these observations the idea has gradually emerged that vascular RLF is a common developmental aberration in infants with immature retinal vessels who breathe air, with or without supplemental oxygen. Moreover, previous preoccupation with the role of oxygen in the production of RLF appears to be giving way to wonder about the complementary observation, i.e., most infants (and all experimental animals) who develop the vascular changes of RLF, even those exposed to high oxygen for prolonged periods, do *not* go on to develop cicatricial changes which produce blindness or retinal scarring (Fig. 9-3). In this connection, the re-awakened interest in evaluation of a protective effect of vitamin E or a potentiating effect of blood transfusion may lead the way to new investigations. Other factors, yet unexplored, may play a role in resisting the effects of oxygen on

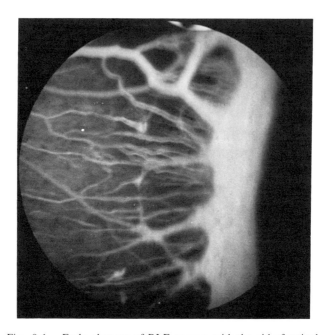

Fig. 9-1. Early changes of RLF as seen with the aid of retinal photography and fluorescein angiography. A *sharp* silver- or gray-appearing abnormal shelf of tissue has formed a border between the central retina (to the left) which has blood vessels and the peripheral portion (to the right) which is devoid of vessels (in contrast to the very gradual change in appearance between these two areas of the retina in the unaffected premature infant). A fluorescein angiogram of the border structure, seen here, reveals that the ledge is a complex of blood vessels in which there is a direct shunt of blood between the arterial and venous circulations.

immature retinal vessels or promoting uncomplicated regrowth after the retinal net of vessels has been obliterated by high oxygen exposure.

New observations and speculations have raised additional doubts about the quick and simple answers of the 1950s to the complex questions concerning oxygen treatment of premature infants. Early mortality among infants in the years before oxygen restriction, during restriction, and in the recent determinative era was reviewed by Cross in 1973 and Bolton and Cross in 1974. From this perspective (Fig. 9-4), the cost of preventing RLF during the period of oxygen restriction was estimated from the decrease in blindness and the rise of day-of-birth deaths during the two decades after the RLF epidemic was brought under control:

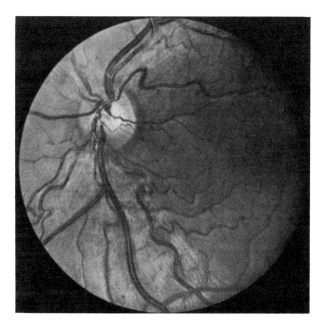

Fig. 9-2. Tortuosity of retinal arteries seen on a photograph of the retina in an ex-premature teenager. Note the hairpin bends in many of the arteries, similar to the changes in the acute vascular stages of RLF during the newborn period (Fig. 1-3, A).

If we say that blindness has fallen from around 50 a year [in England and Wales], and if we say that there has been an excess number of deaths of something over 700 per annum, then it would seem that each sighted baby gained may have cost some 16 deaths.

Although it is impossible to prove the Cross hypothesis, the startling calculation raised the possibility that there is one more blot on the doleful record of the RLF incident. Additionally, the magnitude of "cost" of oxygen restriction in terms of brain damage has not been estimated. For example, it is conceivable that there might be a very small increase in the risk of RLF in contrast to a large reduction in the risk of spastic diplegia (p 56) for infants exposed to continuous supplemental oxygen in concentrations lower than those formally tested in the 1953–54 Cooperative Study. If it should be so, an agonizing reappraisal of the issues involved in oxygen treatment of premature infants would be in order.

The entire matter of long-term outcome in survivors of the RLF epidemic has received relatively little attention from the medical profession.

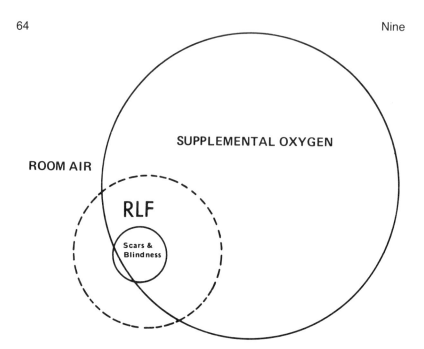

Fig. 9-3. Limitations in the relationship between high oxygen concentration and RLF (acute blood vessel changes—dashed circle; scarring and blindness—small closed circle). Most premature infants exposed to supplemental oxygen do not develop RLF. Some infants who develop RLF have never been exposed to supplemental oxygen.

During the years after the RLF epidemic was "over" for the attendants in premature nurseries (and, later, in intensive care units for the newborn), its impact was in full force (Fig. 9-5) for parents, teachers, social workers, mobility instructors, and others concerned with rehabilitation of the lives of these affected persons. Moreover, there were persistent reports from those with considerable past experience that RLF-blinded children and adults were "different" from other congenitally blind persons. The difference in performance centered around spatial orientation, and the dysfunctions were spotty. For example, the director of an orientation center for the blind told of an RLF-blinded man who played Bach fugues on the piano flawlessly, yet he was unable to replace his shaving razor in its case. When he dropped his towel, he reached up to retrieve it, not down. There have been other anecdotes and allegations of RLF-associated abnormalities but they have never been subjected to intensive investigation. Although the studies in the 1950s of prolonged exposure of newborn animals to oxygen

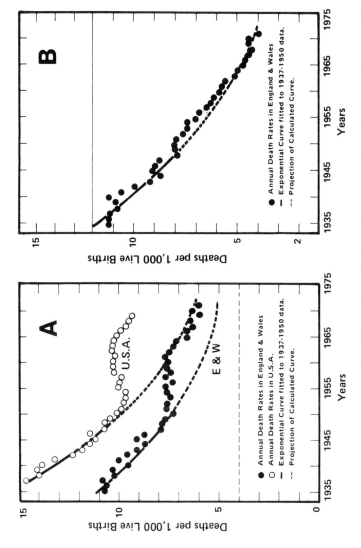

Fig. 9-4. A. In the U.S., England and Wales, *day-of-birth* death rates depart from the projected exponential curves (dashed lines) in the 1950s. The observed death rates began to fall in the mid-1960s but remained displaced from the "expected" line. B. By contrast, death rates in England and Wales for *days-of-life 1–6* show a smooth exponential decline from 1935 through 1970. (See chapter notes for further comments.)

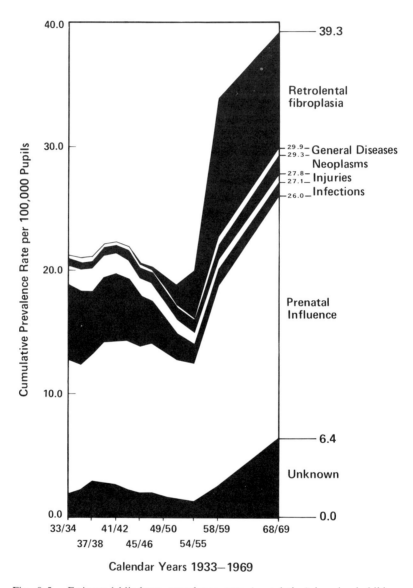

Fig. 9-5. Estimated blindness prevalence rates (cumulative) in school-children by cause in the school years 1933–1934 to 1968–1969.

failed to disclose impressive evidence of gross or microscopic structural changes in the brain, the subject has not been explored exhaustively. Many metabolic reactions in the body are influenced unfavorably by elevated oxygen tension. There is evidence which suggests that the harmful affects are related to the reduction of small amounts of molecular oxygen to transient superoxide free-radicals within the cells of the body. These highly reactive substances produce irreversible damage to vital chemical compounds within cells (enzyme proteins and membrane lipids). In view of earlier observations on the association between iron treatment and RLF (see p 19), it is interesting to note that inorganic iron has a catalytic action which promotes the generation of the potent free-radicals. The potential importance of these considerations to present-day debates concerning the care of newborn infants can be summarized by one question:

Are the eye complications of excessive oxygen the most sensitive endpoints by which to judge a determinative policy of oxygen treatment of premature infants?

10
Medical Inflation

Why did the RLF epidemic begin in the United States in the 1940s? Clues to the answer to this question are to be found, I believe, in some developments which took place immediately after World War II and in the material circumstances of the country during this period. It was an optimistic time in the history of American medicine. When peace was restored, this country, unlike most others, was in a position to direct its attention and considerable resources to deal with medical issues of national importance. Prominent among these was the frequent loss of life among newly born infants. The attack mounted to respond to this challenge in the arena of public health was similar in many ways to the quantitative strategem which brought American victory in the war: mobilization of enormous material assets and rapid increase in technologic development. For the moment I will postpone a discussion about limited strategies in medical "warfare": the slower and safer approaches used in the face of spotty "intelligence". In this chapter I will indicate some of the consequences of the "mass action" approach—how sheer expansion of activities influenced events in American nurseries in the 1940s and 1950s, and I will suggest that the momentum of actions continued to the present time. Some of the elements in this inflation were the increased visibility of premature infants; affluence; proliferation of programs, facilities and equipment; publicity; and the increased influence of authoritative opinion. Some of the disastrous "events" (which I will describe in this chapter) bore a striking resemblance to the RLF prototype.

Innovative effort usually follows closely on the heels of newly visible problems. This relationship was seen in developments which took place in the United States when there was a sharp change in perception of the scope of the topic of premature birth: in 1949, the underdeveloped newborn infant suddenly achieved numerical prominence. Before this time, there was a limited amount of statistical information on prematurity from local areas or from individual hospitals. The Standard Certificate of Live Birth, prior to 1939, did not call for a statement either on the duration of pregnancy or on birth weight. An item on "number of months of pregnancy" was carried on the revised certificate for 1939, but the data obtained were not satisfactory for tabulation. On the 1949 revision of the certificate, the items "Length of pregnancy—weeks" and "Weight at birth" were added. At intervals beginning in 1949, the National Office of Vital Statistics published special reports which indicated that infants weighing less than 2.5 kg (5 lb 8 oz) accounted for a higher toll of infant life than any other condition. The U.S. Children's Bureau presented these data in its publication *Statistical Series* and emphasized the need for concerted action at local, state and national levels. In 1949 the Committee for the Study of Child Health Services of the American Academy of Pediatrics pointed out that in medical schools in the United States training in the care of newborn infants was the weakest feature in the pediatric course and that many teaching hospitals provided very little experience in the care of premature infants. During this same year the U.S. Children's Bureau recommended to the New York Department of Health that the Department of Pediatrics of the New York Hospital–Cornell Medical Center in New York City offer a series of institutes on premature infant care for physicians and nurses. This program of instruction trained physician–nurse teams from many parts of the United States and the instruction model stimulated teaching programs in other areas of the country.

Small babies in the United States also became visible in a literal sense—their clothes were removed. Before the late 1940s, these infants were effectively hidden under layers of swaddling clothes. Only their faces could be seen through single glass doors of incubators with opaque walls (p 44). When the post-war transparent incubators became available (p 48), the new American practice began. (It was theorized that the respiratory movements of a very small infant with a soft rib cage were hampered by heavy clothes and blankets). Nurses and doctors stared at the naked babies as if they were seeing them for the first time. The variations in breathing rhythms recorded with a spirometer in 1942 (p 47) were now visible to the unaided eye. In addition, the outward signs of distressed breathing (indrawing of the chest wall) became evident for the first time. It was found that the respiratory complications of premature infants were very common in the first days of life [especially the respiratory distress syndrome, previously recognized only at post-mortem as hyaline membrane disease (p 54)]. The innocent measure of unwrapping babies exposed them as targets for increased medical actions. The naked infants were examined more completely, observed more closely, and treated more actively than ever before.

Visitors to the United States in the days of the RLF epidemic often voiced the suspicion that American affluence was somehow responsible for the fact that the mysterious affliction occurred most frequently here. In retrospect, the guesses were not far off. American expansion of facilities, on a scale which was beyond the means of many countries, *was* related to the spread of the disorder. Organized programs for specialized care of small babies were developed in some areas of this country before World War II (p 16), but proliferation of specialized centers began during the 1940s. Federal aid for construction of hospital facilities began with the passage of the Hill-Burton Act in 1946. New construction reached a peak in 1949 with completion of the first 1000 projects which received this aid: Hill-Burton funds enabled communities to plan construction of expensive premature infant centers. In 1947, a specialized nursery was opened in Denver at the University of Colorado. It was the focal point of a state-wide program to provide specialized hospital care for premature infants. Another activity of the center was the training of physicians and nurses so that they would be qualified to organize similar projects in other hospitals and communities. In New York City, ten premature centers were established between 1948 and 1953 (the development cost was $2914 per infant bed space). Specialized-bed capacity grew from 52 in 1948 to 303 five years later. An ambulance transport service was established, under the joint administration of the Department of Health and the Department of Hospitals, to transfer babies from the place of birth to the specialized centers (560 infants were transported in the first year of the service; 897 were moved in the fifth year of operation). On July 1, 1950, a payment program was instituted in New York City: costs of care were met by municipal and state funds when parents were unable to pay for specialized care. In 1953, of 2348 babies in centers, 83 percent required full financial assistance. (The average total cost of care for a premature infant in a center, based on an average stay of one month, was $350 during the first 5 years of the program.) North Carolina initiated a program in 1948, and five centers for care of premature infants were opened. Similar programs were developed in other areas; by 1951, three-fourths of states provided some special facilities for the care of premature infants.

Many of the new facilities were designed to provide oxygen from outlets in the wall next to each incubator (piped in from a central source in the hospital). This convenience did away with the frequent and cumbersome task of changing bulky oxygen tanks. Oxygen was now administered continuously, with more ease, and with less conscious attention given to the amount of oxygen consumed—and to cost. The very fact that oxygen was "built-in" provided tacit approval for its free use in American centers.

The spread of costly centers was matched by proliferation of expensive equipment. There was an upsurge of interest in "hardware," now made practical by available funds. In addition to the new Chapple-type incubator (p 48), a number of mechanical contrivances were introduced. One of the earliest was developed in Houston, Texas; the device, called the "Positive Pressure Oxygen–Air Lock" (later, simply "air-lock"), was described in 1950. It was a complicated and expensive machine for resuscitating and oxygenating asphyxiated newborn infants. The apparatus was developed on the basis of the inventor's hypothesis that the newborn infant with respiratory difficulty is managed best by continuing, in so far as possible, the mechanical effects of labor (rhythmic compression of the infant by uterine contractions). The device consisted of a closed chamber in which increased pressures of an oxygen and air mixture were applied to the whole body of the infant occupant. In operation, the "lock" was heated and humidified, the infant was placed in the chamber ventilated by a 60-percent oxygen–air mix, the compartment was sealed and the pressure raised to 2 lb per square inch above atmospheric. The positive pressure was then cycled to 3 lb per square inch over a period of 30–40 seconds; following the "build-up", it was reduced to 1 lb per square inch over a period varying from 15 seconds to as short as 5 seconds. (The pressures used were chosen to mimic the forces on the infant during the most active stage of uterine contractions during labor.) The cycles were repeated at 1-minute intervals until the infant was breathing regularly and skin color was satisfactory; then a steady pressure of 2 lb per square inch of the 60-percent oxygen–air mix was maintained until the infant was removed from the chamber. The initial experience with the device involved 55 infants with respiratory problems who were born in St. Joseph's Maternity Hospital between January 4 and March 26, 1950. Babies remained in the chamber for periods ranging from 1½ to 24 hours; 3 premature infants were in the "lock" for periods of 4–10 days. The death rate of newborn infants in this hospital fell from 1.9 percent the previous year (6324 births) to 1.5 percent (1372 births) in the first 3 months of 1950. The improvement was attributed to the new apparatus and the report concluded that the oxygen–air lock was indicated in any situation requiring oxygenation of newborn infants. Despite many voiced objections concerning the validity of the underlying principles and doubts about the claimed physiologic effects, the device was soon adopted for use in many hospitals throughout the country. Before long, small babies were placed in the lock before symptoms appeared if they were considered to be at risk of developing respiratory distress. Oxygen concentrations above 60 percent were used frequently. When the association between oxygen exposure and RLF was established, there was a strong suspicion that the risk of eye complications was increased at above-atmospheric oxygen pressures. The fear was never substantiated, but use of the air-lock quickly declined. It was largely abandoned even before results of a formal evaluation of the purported life-saving effectiveness of the device were announced in 1956. The early claims of success were not supported: among 72 distressed infants placed in the air-lock for 48 hours, 33 percent succumbed; among 71 in a group of concurrent controls who were not treated with the apparatus, 25 percent died.

The air-lock was followed by a succession of treatment devices (see Table 10-2), but none endured as long as the mist-nebulizer. There were a number of configurations, but all depended on oxygen under pressure (or, less frequently, compressed air) as the propellant force to generate small droplets of water which were blown into infant incubators. Water mist was used to reduce insensible water loss from the body during a period of imposed thirsting after birth (a practice which I will describe shortly). Additionally, nebulized mists were used in the hope of relieving respiratory difficulty by thinning the secretions in the respiratory tract and lung. This approach was given a sharp boost by a startling report from North Carolina, published in 1953. A nebulized mist (using a detergent-like preparation called Alevaire) was claimed as a cure for the respiratory problems of newborn infants! The author cited the favorable experience of others who used the new mist for treatment of various lung conditions in adults and related his own encouraging results in easing the symptoms of older children with respiratory difficulty. This background led him to undertake the treatment of newborn patients. Beginning in April 1951, he placed every infant encountered with symptoms of "asphyxia neonatorum" (a catch-all label for newborn infants with respiratory difficulty) in an incubator filled with detergent-mist. Eighteen small patients were treated: all recovered. This encouraging result was contrasted with a 64-percent mortality among

45 babies with similar symptoms who were treated by other methods in five nearby hospitals. The author concluded the 1953 report of his experience with these words:

It is my considered opinion, after a year's experience, that this is an almost infallible weapon for combatting neonatal asphyxia . . . it enables one to attack this previously discouraging problem with vigor, enthusiasm and confidence . . . one might consider rational, the treatment with [detergent-mist] of all premature babies . . .

The unrestrained language used in this paragraph reveals a good deal about the general outlook of the time, a kind of desire and optimism rolled into one.

In earlier chapters, I traced the origin of the proposals for routine oxygen treatment and in the past few pages I have suggested that the expansion of activities played a role in the increased use of new intensive measures (including the liberal use of oxygen) for the care of premature infants. Now, I wish to emphasize that the changes in caretaking procedures took place in a disjointed manner. The vagaries were related, I believe, to the time-honored empiric approach to clinical problems and to social pressures which encouraged the impatient application of innovations by physicians in the course of their everyday practice. For example, when it became known that "premature infants breathed in a more normal manner in an oxygen-enriched environment" (p 46) and that low oxygen in the blood of these babies could not be detected from outward appearance, (p 46), it seemed entirely reasonable to consider the use of routine oxygen treatment as a corrective measure. The reasoning was sound and physicians responded in predictable fashion. Some said, in effect, Let's try it and see, others indicated, Let's wait and see. I must make it clear that there was no organized campaign to establish a national policy of administering oxygen to all premature infants. Individual activists, and I was among them, jumped from consideration of reasonable theory to application in everyday practice. We crossed the boundary into the unknown quite unconsciously. The move seemed a minor departure from established practice (supplying oxygen only to sick infants) supported by good results reported in Chicago in 1931–33 (p 43). The need for a formal "field" test of the shift to a liberal policy was never considered. This form of optimistic, informal clinical experimentation was customary. Physicians frequently conducted empirical tests of novel and wholly untested treatments in their offices and in hospitals. The results were tabulated after a period of time and reported in statements which began, "In my experience . . ." Moreover, in the immediate post-war period, the spectacular results of newly available treatments (especially penicillin and other new antibiotics for serious infections) encouraged bold explorations. The hope for quick cures was kept alive by news coverage of medical breakthroughs which used the terms "miracie drugs" and "wonder cures." And the spotlight of publicity played an important role in determining the subsequent play of events. This was seen following wide newspaper and magazine coverage of the original article announcing detergent-mist cures; both use and belief spread quickly. Physicians and parents throughout the country were soon clamoring for the new treatment. Interest, hope, and belief were raised to new heights by an article describing the flight of a mercy plane which delivered the detergent preparation to a small hospital for treatment of a desperately ill baby. Following all of the high drama and hyperbole, it was almost impossible to get a fair hearing for the mundane question: Does it really work? In May 1953 we began an evaluation of the new treatment by means of a controlled clinical trial. At the conclusion of the test (which involved 200 infants at Babies Hospital), we were unable to find a beneficial effect of detergent-mist. When these results were published on March 26, 1955, a representative of the company which manufactured the preparation said to me, "It won't hurt our sales." He was right. The negative report had very little effect on the widespread practice. Another formal evaluation of detergent-mist (conducted in Canada) and a trial of the purported beneficial effects of plain water-mist both concluded with similar negative findings. Nonetheless, mist treatment of babies with respiratory symptoms continued for years. Refutations which later appeared inconspicuously in medical journals did little to change the initial judgment made in widely circulated newspaper headlines. Another example of the power of the press to persuade occurred on September 28, 1953. Time Magazine published an article entitled "Too Little and Too Much," which reviewed the subject of RLF. In addition to reporting Campbell's experience (p 26), Time repeated Szewczyk's opinion, that ". . . sudden removal [from oxygen] to normal air may cause retrolental fibroplasia." As a result of this publicity, the "sudden removal" theory achieved a credence which endured for years after evidence to the contrary was published in medical journals.

Following the dramatic events of the first 12 years of the RLF episode, it became obvious that the potential for harm as the result of unrestrained therapeutic exuberance in premature nurseries had become magnified. The expansion of activities and organization of programs throughout the country now involved literally thousands of babies who were treated in new and untested ways; the stakes had been raised considerably. And, the script for potential disaster was outlined in one ordered pattern of action: new proposal—wide application—belated recognition of the possibility of disastrous complications—formal evaluation. The depressing scenario was reenacted in a number of instances which were strikingly similar to that of the RLF incident.

One episode began in 1949, following studies conducted in Boston. It was suggested that many premature infants are born with a surfeit of water and electrolytes in the body. The suggestion was supported by a common observation; the tissues underlying the skin (especially hands and feet) of small newborn babies are often edematous. When fluids and feedings were withheld in a set of planned observations, edematous babies excreted more urine than nonedematous controls. The outward signs of well-being seemed to be satisfactory during the period of thirsting and fasting. Although the blood of these infants became somewhat concentrated, it was shown later that the hemoconcentration could be prevented by placing the babies in incubators filled with water vapor. These observations had important practical implications. The accepted practice of feeding small babies as soon as possible after birth (first with sugar water and, in a few hours, with milk) was always threatened by a feared complication—vomiting and inhalation of the feed into the lungs. If feedings could be withheld safely in the first days, it seemed reasonable to hope that the risk of lung complications from inhalation would be reduced. This reasoning formed the basis for a change in feeding practice which began in the 1950s and quickly spread throughout the United States and, to some extent, abroad. Small infants were placed in incubators saturated with water vapor and all fluids and feedings were withheld until edema in the tissues was no longer evident. The period of initial thirsting and fasting varied from 12 hours to as long as 4 days after birth. The new practice was challenged by Ylppö in Finland (a pioneer in the field of premature infant studies) who argued that premature infants must receive fluid in amounts totalling at least 5 percent of body weight on the first day of life. A controlled trial conducted in Germany in 1955 indicated that premature infants who received early first feedings had a higher survival rate than controls whose feeding was delayed. The European criticism had no influence on the American practice; it continued without serious challenge for more than ten years. In the 1960s, several analytic surveys of past records indicated that brain damage (especially spastic diplegia; see p 56) occurred most frequently among premature infants who had been fasted in the first days of life. By the late 1960s, the thirsting and starving era was over.

Another dramatic shift in feeding practice occurred in the United

States in the 1940s. The change was influenced by studies conducted in New York in 1941 when the premature infant's difficulty in absorbing milk-fat from the intestine was described in quantitative terms. It was found that when human milk or a cow's-milk mixture was fed, a significant fraction of the ingested calories was lost in the stools as unabsorbed fat (Table 10-1). The feeding of half-skimmed milk mixtures resulted in a reduction of fat in the stool. These observations led to a reasonable proposal: if premature infants failed to gain weight on human milk, the calories lost in unabsorbed fat could be reduced by changing the composition of the milk. The proportion of poorly absorbed fat could be reduced, it was suggested, yet the total caloric value of the milk could be maintained by increasing the concentration of well-absorbed protein and carbohydrate. The suggestion was adopted quickly and more generally than originally advised. A half-skimmed cow's-milk mixture was offered from the first feeding; it was not reserved as an alternative for use in infants who failed to gain weight after a trial on human milk. Soon a significant proportion of the (approximately) one-quarter million infants of low birthweight born in the United States each year were receiving a commercial version of the

Table 10-1

Milk Feedings for Premature Infants—Type and
Composition of Feeding, Loss of Calories in Stools

| | | Type of Milk Fed | |
	Human Milk	*Unskimmed Cow's-Milk Mixtures*	*Half-skimmed Cow's-Milk Mixtures*
Fat intake (as percent of caloric intake)*	30–55	30–55	15–20
Protein intake (as percent of caloric intake)*	7	10–20	14–20
Principal type of protein	whey	casein	casein
Loss of calories in stool** (as calories per kg of body weight per day)	ca. 20	ca. 20	ca. 10

*Balance of caloric intake made up of carbohydrate (sugar).
**Unabsorbed milk-fat.

artificial mixture instead of human milk. Not only was the amount of milk-protein increased, but the predominant kind of protein was changed. In cow's milk the principal protein is casein; in human milk whey protein predominates.

There was ongoing debate about this major shift in feeding practice. Although infants fed the artificial-milk mixtures did gain weight relatively rapidly, there was some evidence that much of the increase was accounted for by storage of water and minerals (rather than a primary increase in body tissue). Questions were raised about the burden imposed on body metabolism if more protein was absorbed than could be utilized in the formation of tissues of fixed protein composition. The speculation was not idle. Small babies who received high-protein feedings had elevated concentrations of a protein metabolite (the amino acid tyrosine) in the blood during the first days of life. Since this amino acid was thought to be capable of injuring the developing brain, fears arose, but the practice continued. Debate about the possibility of brain damage went on for years. It was not silenced by follow-up surveys conducted in the 1960s which were unable to demonstrate an increased frequency of neurologic complications. In the past few years, additional suspicions concerning the safety of feeding cow's milk have been raised. The intensity of the debate has increased as a number of metabolic changes have been measured which appear to be related to the quantity and to the quality of protein fed to premature infants.

In the 1970s studies conducted in Finland in collaboration with an American group suggested that prematurely born infants have a limited capacity to make taurine (a free amino acid which is not incorporated into protein; there is evidence that it is important to normal function of the retina and to normal development of the brain). In carefully designed randomized feeding trials, the Finnish-American study demonstrated that infants fed casein-predominant milk preparations (which contain virtually no taurine) had very much lower amounts of this substance in their blood and urine than was found in concurrent controls who received human milk (a rich source of taurine). The findings suggested that the rapidly growing premature infant may be dependent on a dietary source for this essential material. Although the effects of the long-standing practice of feeding premature infants low-taurine milk mixtures are unknown, studies of taurine deficiency in other species have revealed some disturbing results. For example, in the cat, taurine deficiency is associated with degeneration of the retina; blindness results if dietary taurine is not supplied. These dire speculations and other studies of non-nutritive advantages of human milk for premature infants have been responsible for recent increased interest in a return to use of mother's milk in this country. The order of events which I have just described resemble the sequence associated with shifts in oxygen treatment practices in the same American nurseries. Widespread change took place quickly; "field" testing (if it occurred at all) followed far behind.

The hapless scenario was not confined to slowly evolving events in which unexpected complications were difficult to detect (the changes in the eyes seen weeks after oxygen treatment was stopped, or signs of neurologic handicap detected years after a period of initial fasting in the first days of life). During the 1950s, there were several treatment catastrophes in which the outward signs of serious complications occurred immediately. The time scale was compressed, but the script resembled that of the RLF saga. The first of these incidents originated in a change in opinion/practice which occurred between 1947 and 1949. For a few years prior to this time, bacterial infections, when they were identified in premature infants, were treated with the post-World War II "miracle" drugs (sulfonamides and penicillin), but results were quite poor. The principal difficulty seemed to be the vague nature of early signs of serious infection in small babies. Diagnosis was often delayed or missed entirely. In 1947, a new approach to this problem was proposed in Edinburgh, Scotland: penicillin was administered for the first week of life to *all* infants who weighed less than 1.6 kg (3 lb 9 oz). An improvement in survival rate was reported. A similar experience was reported in 1949 from Mälmo, Sweden following the use of penicillin and sulfanilamides. The practice of routine administration of antibacterial drugs was not widely used in Europe, but it was quickly adopted in the United States. At the annual meeting of the American Pediatric Society in 1949, a leading authority from Boston recommended a number of measures for the prevention and control of infections in newborn infants. Among the suggestions, he advised, "In nurseries for premature infants outside [of] obstetric hospitals, all infants, with the possible exception of healthy newborn infants, should be given a prophylactic course of treatment with sulfadiazine and penicillin." He noted that, "The vital statistics from this nursery for 1948 show a dramatic reduction in mortality for all infants weighing 2 kg (4 lb 7 oz) or less." In the discussion of this report, a commentator from Denver said, ". . . we use sulfadiazine and antibiotics freely." When the premature center at Babies Hospital in New York opened in late 1949, the new practice suggested at the annual meeting was adopted. Antibacterial drugs (penicillin plus oxytetracycline or chloramphenicol) were administered to all infants transferred-in from other hospitals in the hope of reducing the risk of outbreaks of infection which might be "imported" from other nurseries. This routine continued for 3½ years. In 1953, a new combination of drugs for prevention was considered: penicillin plus a newly available sulfonamide drug (sulfisoxazole). The new agent had a practical advantage over previous preparations; it could be administered by injection at infrequent intervals (once or twice each day to maintain satisfactory levels in the blood). The new regimen was prescribed at Babies Hospital for 1½ years with no recognized hint of difficulty. The mortality rate of very small infants was quite high in the early 1950s. The deaths were associated with a number of fatal conditions (especially hyaline membrane disease— p 54), and kernicterus, a damaging, often fatal form of brain damage which is a complication of jaundice in new born infants). But, "in our experience . . ." the frequency of fatal infections was relatively low in association with the preventive treatment.

When the results of the RLF Cooperative Trial became known in 1954, our skepticism concerning all unevaluated innovations in premature care began to grow. A recommendation for a new antibacterial treatment program was made in that year, and we seized on the opportunity to begin a long-delayed systematic examination of this element of care. At this time, we thought the grounds for recommending preventive treatment were quite reasonable; only the ideal agent(s) seemed in doubt. Consequently, we decided to compare the results of the proposed new treatment (subcutaneous oxytetracycline) with those of the "established" drugs (penicillin plus sulfisoxazole). We were completely unprepared for the denouement at the end of this exercise. We anticipated the controlled trial would be the first in a series of exploratory attempts to find an ideal preventive regimen. It seemed unlikely the differences would be striking and we thought we were in for a long search. Much to our amazement, the first trial gave a definitive result. To our horror, the mortality rate was highest (and strikingly so) in infants who received the "established" treatment! Infants who received penicillin plus sulfisoxazole had fewer infections, as compared with the babies who received the new treatment, but this was irrelevant. Kernicterus was found nine times more often among infants who succumbed after receiving the standard treatment. There was little doubt that this unexpected (and, at the time, completely inexplicable) complication accounted for the increased number of fatalities. We took little comfort in the undeniable fact that the formal trial "saved" half of the infants from exposure to the unsuspected hazards of a treatment which had been used so confidently for the previous 1½ years. If a controlled trial had been carried out at the time of the original shift in practice, the "saving" in lives would have been truly impressive. It was not until 1959 that the mechanism underlying the disaster was uncovered. It was found that sulfonamide drugs (especially sulfisoxazole) "released" the yellow pigment bilirubin from its binding to albumin in the blood of jaundiced infants; the toxic pigment was then free to enter the brain. Since sulfonamide drugs were used widely in the treatment of newborn infants (many of whom were jaundiced), this fatal complication must have occurred often. However, the national dimensions of the kernicterus outbreak were never reported.

The deep-seated perseverance of the custom of informal experimentation in medicine is illustrated vividly by an incident which occurred while the lessons of the RLF and the kernicterus outbreaks were still ringing in the ears of pediatricians. The episode began one quiet Saturday afternoon in 1956. Ethel Dunham, who was revising her textbook *(Premature Infants),* came to New York to ask my colleague, Hattie Alexander of Columbia University, about the subject of antibacterial treatment. Doctor Alexander was a renowned authority on the subject of infectious disease. She was disturbed by the very poor experience in treating the class of infections caused by coliform bacteria. These infections were becoming prominent in newborn infants, as others caused by organisms which responded to penicillin were subsiding. Mindful of the recent kernicterus disaster in our nursery, she told Doctor Dunham that new steps must be taken cautiously. Doctor Alexander proposed that a controlled clinical trial be conducted to explore the effectiveness of a combination of agents in infants at highest risk [those weighing under 2 kg (4 lb 7 oz) at birth]. Shortly afterward, at a seminar on premature infants which Doctor Richard L. Day and I coordinated, Doctor Alexander gave a short talk on antibacterial therapy and announced her proposal in these words:

> . . . the following combination of antibiotic agents would be worthy of trial
> . . . [in] all infants whose birth weights are less than 2000 grams:
> 1. Chloramphenicol
> 2. Erythromycin
> 3. Sulfadiazine

(The dose of chloramphenicol recommended was 100 mg per kilogram per day, the dose used in older infants and children). This talk, in a small parlor room of the Biltmore Hotel in midtown Manhattan on October 7, 1956, was the only time that the proposal was ever made publicly (the report of the seminar did not appear in print until 9 months later). Despite the express recommendation for an evaluative trial, the caution was not heeded. Instead, uncontrolled use of the suggested treatment regimen (and other variations using chloramphenicol) spread quickly to all of the states of the Union. The sorrowful consequences slowly became evident in the next few years. In all parts of the country, nurses and physicians observed a strange new disorder of premature infants. It came to be known as the "gray syndrome": on the third or fourth day of life, the babies developed distention of the abdomen, vomiting, irregular respirations, and pallor. Cyanosis and poor circulation of blood to the peripheral tissues quickly followed and the victims developed a ghastly gray color of the skin. In a few hours, they were dead. During these years there were several severe influenza epidemics in the United States; deaths from pneumonia occurred frequently in the nurseries. As a result, it was some time before the association was made between the new drug treatment of infections and the horrendous gray syndrome. All doubt ended in 1959, when the results of a controlled clinical trial, conducted in Los Angeles, were reported: the mortality rate among infants who received chloramphenicol was substantially higher than in untreated concurrent controls. It was found, belatedly, that premature infants have a limited ability to transform and to excrete chloramphenicol. The relatively high doses administered resulted in fatally high levels of drug in the blood.

What stands out in this review of calamities (and there were other similar episodes) is unrestrained medical behavior: a double standard of evidence was used to guide actions. In preclinical investigations involving animals or in pilot observations in infants, the rules of scientific evidence were carefully observed. At the next step in investigation, the first application of new treatment in the "field," the cautious rules were abandoned. The safeguards inherent in the hedging strategy of formal evaluation (limited exposure of infants to unknown risks through use of controls) were exploited as an afterthought. Over and over, the barn door was locked after the horse had escaped!

On one occasion, the "door" was locked *just* as the "horse" was escaping. This incident began with a drug company application to the Food and Drug Administration on September 16, 1960, for distribution of a new drug in the United States. The drug, thalidomide, had been in general use in West Germany since 1957: it was well regarded there as a safe and useful medication, especially in the treatment of nausea in pregnancy. The company was required to present the results of clinical testing in this country before F.D.A. approval was granted. To meet this requirement, the firm sent 2.5 million tablets to 1267 "investigators" in the United States. However, it was clear that no formal studies were expected. A manual issued to salesmen employed by the company stated, ". . . the main purpose is to establish local studies whose results will be spread among hospital members. You can assure your doctors that they need not report results if they don't want to . . ." At this time, and quite by chance, Doctor Frances Kelsey, of the F.D.A., read a short letter to the editor in the British Medical Journal of December 31, 1960. The letter mentioned the possibility that use of thalidomide might result in certain neurologic symptoms in the feet and hands (peripheral neuritis) of adult users. Alerted by this suggestion, Doctor Kelsey began to request more information concerning the complication from the company. On February 23, 1961 she requested a complete list of investigators to whom the drug had been furnished, hoping to check on possible neurologic effects. The company sent a list of only 56 investigators who had used the drug for a period of 4 months or longer. Little by little it was learned that thalidomide taken by pregnant women was the suspected cause of congenital malformations. As early as October 1960, the first two cases of grossly deformed babies (with seal-like deformities of the limbs) were presented at a medical exhibit in West Germany. In late 1961, the West German Minister of Health issued a statement warning women not to take the drug. Finally, thalidomide was withdrawn from the market in West Germany on November 25, 1961. Following this action, reports from country after country indicated that thousands of malformed babies had been affected.

The drug never emerged out of investigational status in the United States, thanks to the actions of Doctor Kelsey. Later the F.D.A. conducted an inquiry which revealed that hundreds of the "investigators" who received the drug for study in this country failed to keep adequate records. They did not know which patients received the drug, nor when it was prescribed and at what dosage. When the hazards became known, the F.D.A. investigators were unable to contact many of the patients. More than half of 1258 physicians interviewed had no record of the quantities of the drug returned or destroyed, pursuant to the manufacturer's instructions.

Legislative recognition of this situation came with the passage of the Kefauver-Harris Amendment to the U.S. Pure Food and Drug Laws in 1962. For the first time, there were legal regulations governing the formal and limited steps taken in testing the safety and efficacy of a new drug for use in human patients. Unfortunately, this law, and subsequent F.D.A. regulations, have not provided adequate protection for the fetus and newborn infant. Only rarely are the controlled testing programs carried out in these immature patients (whose metabolism of drugs is frequently quite different from that seen in older individuals). Moreover, many informal clinical investigations (involving drugs which are not "approved" for use in the fetus and newborn, and physical maneuvers which do not involve drugs) are still carried out in the casual style which characterized thalidomide "investigations" in this country. As late as 1972, one leader in perinatal medicine said:

Therapeutic programs which evolve are difficult to subject to controlled studies, particularly when they appear to be successful . . . I think in some instances, gradual change in therapy often leads to sounder practice . . .

Unfortunately, the results of most "gradual changes in therapy" that have taken place in the evolvement of modern perinatal medicine do not bear out this optimism (Table 10-2).

The phrase "gradual change in therapy" conjures up an image of slow, cautious exploration, but is this accurate? I said earlier that there was a Let's-wait-and-see response from some physicians when they first learned about the reasoned suggestions for routine oxygen treatment. At the 1949 meeting, when routine antibacterial drug treatment was advised, one commentator said "I am disturbed at . . . [the] advocacy of routine treatment with penicillin and sulfadiazine for all babies. Would not more difficulty arise from that procedure in the long run?" What converted the doubters? It was not, as I have shown, the presentation of reliable evidence from formal trials; there were few die-hards who waited that long. Moreover, the conversions took place so quickly that it seems likely some social forces were at work. A sociologic study, reported in 1957, of the diffusion of a innovation among physicians provides a number of insights into the dynamics of the conversion process: the propagation of "fashions" in therapy.

Coleman and co-workers examined the social influences which intervened between the initial prescription of a new drug by a few innovators and its final use by virtually an entire medical community. Data were collected in four American cities for 15 months after a new antibiotic drug with wide potential applicability was released for general use. The researchers conducted sociometric interviews and classified 125 physicians, on the basis of individual attributes, into two mutually exclusive classes: primarily physician-oriented (principally on the basis of recognition given by colleagues) or primarily patient-oriented (respect by patients and general standing in the community). In addition, they traced the social structure which linked the doctors together: professional relationships (advisors and discussion partners) and friendship ties. The month when each physician first prescribed the drug was determined by systematic monitoring of the prescription records of pharmacies in the cities over the period of study. Coleman's group found that physician-oriented doctors generally used the

Table 10-2

Results of some "Proclaimed" Therapies in the
Development of Perinatal Medicine

Gradual Changes in Therapy	Consequences*		
	Led to Sounder Practice	*Led to Disaster*	*Misled into Fruitless Byways*
Testosterone to stimulate growth of prematures		?	
Thyroid hormone . . ibid . . .			×
DES to prevent miscarriage		×	
Progestins to prevent miscarriage		×	
Exchange transfusion	×		
Supplemental oxygen for periodic breathing		×	
Initial thirsting and starving		× (?)	
Synthetic vitamin K prophylaxis		×	
Low-fat, high-protein feedings		?	
Sulfisoxazole prophylaxis		×	
Chloramphenicol prophylaxis		×	
Gastric emptying to prevent RDS**			×
Sternal traction for RDS			×
Epsom salt enemas for RDS		×	
Rocking-bed for RDS			×
Alevaire for RDS			×
Water mist for RDS			×
Acetylcholine for RDS			×
Respirator support in RDS	×		
Continuous positive airway pressure for RDS	× (?)		
Feeding gastrostomy for prematures		?	×
Ice water resuscitation for asphyxia			×
Sodium bicarbonate bolus infusions in asphyxia	?		
Lowered thermal environment		×	
Routine hexachlorophene bathing		?	
Phototherapy for hyperbilirubinemia	× (?)		

*Most of these judgements rest on as infirm a base as the original claims of benefit (see chapter notes).

**Respiratory distress syndrome (see p 54).

drug earlier than their patient-oriented colleagues. However, a plot of the curve of cumulative proportion of new users had the same shape in both groups (the curve for the patient-oriented physicians was merely displaced to later starting times). In both groups the movement resembled a "snow-ball" process: the number of recruits each month increased in proportion to those who were already converted. (The mathematical equation of this curve characterizes rates of population growth, certain chemical reactions, and other phenomena which obey a chain-reaction process.) Additionally, there appeared to be successive stages in which interpersonal influences played a role in diffusion of the innovation through the community of physicians. The first social networks which appeared to be influential were those which connect doctors in professional relationships of advisors and discussion partners. A little later the friendship ties seemed to exert a persuasive influence. Finally, by about 6 months after the drug was re-leased, the social networks seemed completely inoperative as chains of influence. Early, when a minority of physicians were prescribing the drug, intellectual assurance from esteemed colleagues and emotional support from friends seemed to be needed by those who were uncertain. As the "snow-ball" process gathered momentum, usage was no longer novel and late recruits turned less and less to individuals for validation and approval.

The Coleman group observations suggest that advisors play a pivotal role in the initial phase of the diffusion of an innovation. This was borne out in the shift to routine oxygen treatment in the 1940s. Early adoption of the new practice took place in the leading (physician-oriented) university hospitals in the United States. I can recall enactment of the advisor role when the routine was just beginning in New York. Doctors from small hospitals visited Columbia University and asked not only about the ration-ale for the shift, but they also wanted to know if this was occurring in other prestigious institutions. Before long, routine oxygen was used so widely that the questions stopped. Acceptance of this "fashion" in treatment was complete.

The speed of propagation of information about treatment "fashions" has increased considerably since the days of mist treatment in 1953 and the Coleman study in the mid-1950s. Physicians and the public are bombarded with medical news in print media (and, of course, television). Physicians receive additional information in the form of digests and summaries of original reports and of lectures. These appear in medical newspapers and magazines which are sent free of charge to doctors (the number of these drug-advertisement-supported publications has increased considerably since the 1950s). As a result of the profusion of medical news reporting, it is increasingly probable that a physician will first learn about a new treatment from some secondary source—an abbreviated account that does not present all of the evidence, nor the details of the design of studies on which the conclusions are based. Furthermore, encouraging, positive results are reported in the news more frequently than failures. For example, an article appeared on page 1 of the New York Times on October 22, 1964 under the headline "Fatal Baby Disease is Reported Cured." The information was obtained from a talk delivered the day before in Miami, Florida to an audience of physicians attending the annual meeting of the College of American Pathologists and the American Society of Clinical Pathologists. The story began, "A cure for the mysterious hyaline membrane disease, which takes the lives of up to 25,000 infants in the United States each year, was reported here today [October 21] at a medical meeting. A little more than a year ago the disease was fatal to Patrick Bouvier Kennedy, infant son of President Kennedy." The reporter explained that a new treatment had been devised based on the idea that newborns have too much water in their bodies; in prematures, in particular, excretion of water by the immature kidney is impaired. Water tries to escape through the incompletely developed lungs, he continued; this chokes off the air supply, leading to the symptoms of respiratory distress and death. The simple new theory led to a simple new treatment: enemas of saturated epsom salts immediately after birth to draw off water from the body tissues. "It is not yet certain that the theory is correct," the reporter noted, "but it is certain that the treatment works." The concentrated enemas were given to 28 sick infants in five hospitals in Louisville, Kentucky; all 28 improved dramatically. Babies who were suffocating became "normal" in an hour or less. The New York Times reporter interviewed the originator of the enema treatment and he relayed the suggestion that ". . . all premature infants be given the treatment prophylactically [since] it cannot be determined which infants will develop the disease . . . and the treatment itself appears to be without hazard. Prophylactic use of epsom-salt enemas will prevent the development of the disease and save many lives." This news was reported extensively in general news media (including Time Magazine on Oct. 30, 1964) and in the medical news publications (including Medical Tribune on November 11, 1964). Even the highly respected Lancet carried an annotation (November 21, 1964) which began, "A new treatment for premature infants with hyaline-membrane disease was suggested at a meeting . . . last month . . . the full details have not yet reached us . . .," and the editor went on to describe the available facts gleaned from the New York Times article. The news stories were much more efficient than the doctor-to-doctor grapevine: use of enemas spread more quickly than did prescriptions of chloramphenicol 8 years earlier—and the denouement came more quickly. On July 5, 1965, Andrews and his associates reported the results of magnesium sulfate (epsom salt) enemas given to 10 newborn lambs: concentrated solutions were uniformly fatal (5 lambs who received 50-percent-solution enemas developed elevated levels of magnesium in the blood, signs of magnesium intoxication, and all died 23–46 minutes later), and less concentrated solutions also produced disturbing results (2 of 5 lambs receiving 25-percent-solution enemas developed signs of magnesium intoxication; 1 died 2 hours later). Needless to say, these alarming observations had a chilling effect. Use of the outlandish treatment fell off sharply, but not completely. Seven years after the results in lambs were reported, it was still found necessary to publish a warning against the dangers of the epsom-salt enemas (an instance had been encountered of fatal magnesium intoxication following an enema treatment for hyaline membrane disease). Unfortunately, the story of the incredible epsom-salt enemas is not unusual. Once brought to life by press attention, even the most bizarre treatment (Laetrile treatment for cancer is a notorious example, see chapter notes) may lead a hydra-like existence.

Roger Bacon, in the 13th century, warned against uncritical acceptance of authoritative opinion, but it was still a major stumbling block in medicine during the years which I have recalled in this chapter. Unhappily, skepticism has fallen even lower in the years since. Physicians depend, more than ever, on the judgments and opinions of authorities because of an exponential increase in scientific information and an increase in the complexity of medicine. At the same time the voice of authority is louder and more broadly cast than ever: the electronic revolution carries the voice of experts and the jet airplane carries the experts themselves into every corner of the country. The potential for misinterpretation of the kind which took place in that small hotel room in 1956 (concerning chloramphenicol) is now enormous. Moreover, more attention is paid to the speaker than to the content of his remarks. Objective evidence of this "personalization" phenomenon was obtained by Naftulin and co-workers. They framed the following hypothesis: given an impressive lecturer and lecture format, even an experienced group of listeners (professional medical educators) will be seduced into feeling they have learned something—even when the content of the lecture has been irrelevant, conflicting, and meaningless. A distinguished-appearing, authoritative-sounding professional actor was dubbed "Doctor Myron L. Fox" and given impressive but fictitious credentials. He spoke to several important audiences on "Mathematical Game Theory as Applied to

Physician Education.'' The lectures and the question-and-answer sessions were filled with double-talk, neologisms, *non sequiturs,* contradictory statements, meaningless references to unrelated topics—and some good jokes. Satisfaction questionnaires returned by the audiences gave the lecture a high rating. The phenomenon has been labeled "The Doctor Fox Effect" and it deserves special recognition. It raises an issue concerning the responsibility of authorities who speak to practicing physicians, and more so when their remarks are reported in the press. If authoritative statements are accepted completely uncritically, lecturers have an incommutable obligation to use restraint and self-criticism. The duty is particularly great when speaking about unevaluated innovations to physicians who are pressed to find solutions to their everyday medical problems. Authoritative lecturers should stimulate their listeners to responsible contemplation of incomplete evidence, instead of irresponsible, unrestrained action. The disturbing consequences of impatient action which I have reviewed recall an apocryphal saying in factories which manufacture fireworks:

It is better to curse the darkness, than to light the wrong candle.

11
The Price of Progress

I have focused so closely on the treatment disasters which occurred during the first decades after World War II that I must declare the obvious: the picture was not one of unrelieved gloom. New knowledge resulting from expanded preclinical research gave rise to clinical applications which seem to have passed the crude test of time (although there is no way of knowing whether all of the "ticking bombs" have been detected). There has been resigned, almost philosophic, acceptance (in the medical community and in the community-at-large) of the view that the "accidents" which occurred were the inevitable price that had to be paid for progress. Public support for clinical explorations was whole-hearted in the early years. The success of the Cooperative Study of RLF in ending the blindness epidemic was often mentioned in news accounts as an example (and, in 1953, one of the earliest instances) of the effective use of government monies for extramural clinical research (research not performed *directly* by federal agencies). The visible return of government investment in the 1954 field trial of the Salk poliomyelitis vaccine—the largest public health experiment ever conducted —added to public awareness and approval. In the late 1950s, requests to Congress for funds to expand the National Institutes of Health extramural research programs (both preclinical and clinical) cited the conquests of RLF and polio as bread-cast-upon-the-water examples. Congress was lavish in its praises and largesse. In the 5-year period between 1955 and 1960, a great deal of federal "bread" was cast into the medical ocean (Table 11-1).

Table 11-1

National Institutes of Health Research Grant Expenditures and
U.S. Gross National Product in 1950, 1955 and 1960*

Calendar Year	N.I.H. Research Grant Expenditure (in millions)	Gross National Product (in billions)	Research Grants As Proportion of GNP[a]
1950	$ 15.0	$284.8	$ 52,700
1955	35.5	398.0	89,200[b]
1960	198.8	503.7	394,700[c]

*See chapter notes.

[a]Research grants as dollars per billion dollars GNP.

[b]Research grants as proportion of GNP rose 69 percent from 1950 to 1955.

[c]Research grants as proportion of GNP rose 342 percent from 1955 to 1960.

The large disbursements spurred development of the programs for premature infant care which were described in Chapter 10. At the same time, research activities which were directed at neonatal and, later, prenatal problems expanded remarkably in the United States and abroad following the RLF incident (Table 11-2). There was intensification of background studies in physiology and biochemistry. Knowledge concerning perinatal matters increased immeasurably, and the momentum has continued to the present day. Developments and innovations in the management of pregnancy have been extended and elaborated to include evaluation of the well-being of the fetus. Care of the new infant now begins well before birth. The

Table 11-2

Citations Concerned with Perinatal Topics and Total Medical
Citations in 1950, 1955 and 1960

Calendar Year	Perinatal Citations[a]	Total Citations[b]	Perinatal Citations as Proportion of Total (per 1000)
1950	453	ca. 92,500	ca. 5
1955	652[c]	ca. 107,500	ca. 6
1960	1373[d]	ca. 125,000	ca. 11[e]

[a]Citations under the headings Fetus; Infant, newborn; and Infant, premature (see chapter notes).

[b]These are approximations (i.e. number of pages × average number of citations per page—see chapter notes).

[c]The number of perinatal citations rose 44 percent between 1950 and 1955.

[d]The number of perinatal citations rose 111 percent between 1955 and 1960.

[e]The proportion of perinatal citations rose about 83 percent between 1955 and 1960.

state of health of the fetus can be assessed from measurements in mother's blood and urine and from small samples of amniotic fluid (obtained by amniocentesis). Genetic defects (and the gender of the fetus) may be determined early in pregnancy by examining cells in amniotic fluid and by chemical analyses of the fluid. The growth of the fetus (especially the head) can be measured accurately by means of serial ultrasound images. The position and function of the supply organ of the fetus—the placenta—can be monitored. The state of maturation of the lung (which determines the risk of developing hyaline-membrane disease) can be assessed from chemical analysis in amniotic fluid, and lung maturation can be accelerated [by administering a hormonal drug (betamethasone) to the mother] when premature delivery is threatened. During labor and delivery the fetal heart rate can be monitored continuously and, from samples of blood taken from the scalp of the fetus, the biochemical status (acid–base and blood gases) can be accurately gauged. After delivery, electronic and biochemical surveillance of the small and sick newborn infant take place in intensive care units under the supervision of highly trained personnel and with the help of all of the panoply of modern life-support "hardware."

From the "inevitable-accidents-as-the-price-of-progress" point of view, the costs of the misadventures along the way must be weighed in the balance. It can be argued that the net gains for American infants have been enormous because of the expansion of activities brought about by the investment of public funds in perinatal research since the mid-1950s. For proof, according to this view, one has only to point to the progressive improvement in outcome of pregnancy and delivery, as measured by intact survival. The same general argument has been made concerning the beneficial effect of expansions in all other fields of modern medicine. And, the formulation has been subjected to increasing criticism from many quarters in recent years. The debates are timely, and, in my opinion, will lead to long-overdue inspection of some fixed dogmas. For example, the "inevitability-of-accidents" premise deserves a close look, and I shall return to a criticism of this belief in the chapters which follow. At this point I wish to take issue with the other propositions in the argument.

First, the conventional opinion concerning the immediacy of the growth of modern scientific medicine should not be allowed to pass without a challenge. There is some evidence which suggests that this perspective of the recent past may be much too narrow. Price calculated the rate of growth of science as a whole (using numbers of publications and the size of scientific manpower as quantitative indicators). He found that the present exponential rate has been steady for some time:

In 1900, in 1800 and perhaps 1700, one could look back and say that the number of scientists alive is greater than the total number of all previous scientists and most of what is known . . . has been determined within living memory. Scientists have always felt themselves to be awash in a sea of scientific literature that augments in each decade as much as in all times before.

The popular view that the advancement of medical knowledge is solely the result of increased expenditure of public funds for medical research (the notion that new ideas can be purchased) is a worrisome distortion of reality. Indeed, there is reason to suspect, from Price's studies, that the gains from increased expenditure are limited by the law of diminishing returns. He found an inflationary trend (in science as a whole) during the past few decades in the United States, the U.S.S.R., and less so in the rest of the world. With the marked increase in social status of the scientist and need for his services, competition developed: general salaries rose, and there were automatic increases in research funds and facilities commanded by the prestige and by the cargo cult of modern science. Each increase in prestige produced a pay-off in increased scientific results, but heightened competition raised the stakes for the next round. A recent critique of Soviet science also raised questions about the quality of research as volume increased. One Russian scientist opined, "You can't make an ocean liner by stringing together a bunch of row boats."

Additionally, the *post hoc* argument which implies that most of the improvement in medical outcomes (particularly in perinatal results) in the United States is the result of specific technical interventions overstates the case for causality. In spite of the solidly grounded scientific studies on which many of the present-day developments in perinatal medicine are based, there have been few systematic attempts to evaluate their practical effects. The relative contribution of the technical inflation to secular trends in perinatal mortality rates is unknown. The "in-tandem" effects of social and demographic changes which have occurred in the United States cannot be ignored. For example, significant changes in the distributions of births occurred when there was an overall decline in birth rate in New York City (following the establishment of widely available family-planning services in the years 1966–1970, and legalized abortion beginning in 1970). The fall-off in rates of birth among "high-risk" groups (women whose risk of premature birth was known to be high were they to become pregnant) was particularly abrupt; these groups were

—women at both extremes of the childbearing age-range (the very young and the relatively older women);

—women who had a history of many births;
—unmarried women;
—women whose socioeconomic status was relatively low.

And, there was a marked decline in the births of small babies, especially those weighing 1.5 kg (= 3 lb 5 oz) or less. These shifts were accompanied by an unprecedented fall in infant mortality (the decrease was particularly striking in the years following legalized abortion). A similar experience was reported by Lee and others at Bronx Municipal Center in New York City. They analyzed mortalities which occurred among newborns in this hospital during the years 1966 through 1973. There was a close relationship between annual mortality rate and the proportion of very-low-birth-weight babies (under 1.5 kg) born each year. In 1970, two events occurred: intensive care of newborn infants was increased at the hospital (there were significant changes in trained personnel and introduction of specialized equipment), and an active abortion program was initiated. Analysis of the fall in mortality rates which occurred in the unit in the years following the two changes suggested that a relatively steep reduction in the births of very small babies accounted for three-quarters of the improvement; the remaining difference could be attributed either to improved medical care or to improved health status of the infants at birth.

Morris and coworkers evaluated several possible causes for the decline in infant mortality seen throughout the United States during the late 1960s. They found a systematic shift in the distribution of births during this period from relatively high-risk categories to those of lower risk for infant mortality (Fig. 11-1). The changing maternal-age/birth-order distribution of births since 1965 accounted for about 27 percent of the reduction in infant mortality rate that occurred over the next 12 years in the United States. The contribution of organized Maternal and Infant Care Projects (funded by the U.S. Children's Bureau beginning in 1965) was also examined. Under the most generous assumptions, only a small fraction of the decline in mortality could possibly be attributed to the success of this well-intentioned effort to deliver high-quality services to high-risk mothers and infants. From other (sporadic) studies, there is reason to suspect that other factors (e.g., increased use of contraception for spacing pregnancies, increased economic and social support during pregnancy, increased emphasis on the importance of adequate diet in pregnancy) also may have contributed to the changes in pregnancy outcome in recent years.

Despite the continuing trend of decreased mortality rates, the United States, as it has for many years, has a relatively low standing in interna-

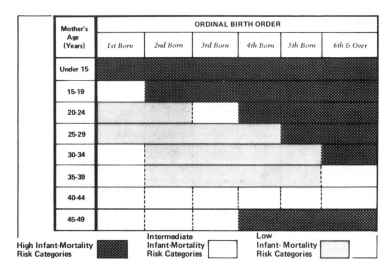

Fig. 11-1. Infant-mortality risk categories by mother's age at different ordinal numbers-of-birth. Beginning in 1965 (through 1972), a shift occurred in the distribution of births in the United States: from the high-risk age/birth-order categories toward the low-risk "cells." This shift was sufficient to account for about 27 percent of the reduction in U.S. infant mortality.

tional comparisons. The lag is frequently quoted in support of the need for increased supply of personnel, facilities and equipment for intensive technical supervision of perinatal activities. In this connection, Hinds examined the relationship between infant mortality rate and the number of health care workers available (per capita) for the years 1966 through 1970 in 28 developed countries of North America, Europe, Asia, and Oceania. Lower rates of mortality were more closely related to numbers of auxilliary health workers (nurses and midwives) than to the numbers of physicians available. St. Leger also explored the relationship between infant mortality and the provision of doctors (making an adjustment for the variations in affluence in 18 developed countries, as measured by gross national product per capita—Fig. 11-2). The strong positive correlation seen in his figure (countries with the greatest number of physicians per capita had the highest infant mortality) is just as provocative (and as suspect) as the oft-cited relationship between increased technical interventions and survival.

There are also questions about the relationship between interventions and the "quality" of survival. A community study conducted in Newcastle upon Tyne, England, recorded the functional abilities in the first decade of

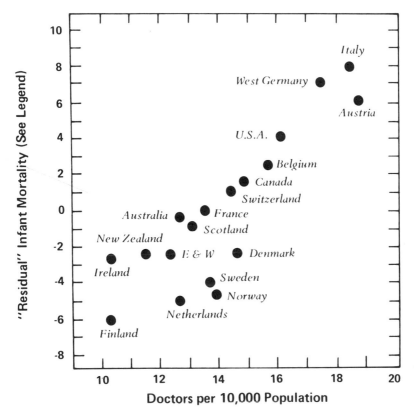

Fig. 11-2. Relationship between infant mortality and doctors provided per 10,000 population in 18 developed countries examined by St. Leger. Mortality is expressed as the "residual" difference after making an allowance for gross national product per capita in these countries (1970 data).

life of 13,203 children born in the years 1960 through 1962. It was found that even two of the most lethal perinatal adverse factors which can be directly modified by medical actions (breech delivery and prolonged delay in establishing regular respiration) appeared to have only trivial effects on the subsequent neurologic state of the children. Any effects which they may have had on the intelligence or the behavior of the survivors were explained by an association with two groups of much more potent determinants: biologic characteristics and social factors. In the first category, variations in birth weight seemed to have the most important effect: low birthweight was the characteristic most commonly associated with recognizable forms of brain damage. The second group of factors, whose effects far outweighed those of the perinatal ones, comprised the social attributes. The least specific, and yet the most powerful of these, was the child's social class of origin as determined by father's occupation. The cultural and general environmental implications of social class appeared to be of paramount importance in determining outcome. In a large U.S. study, the perinatal correlates of intellectual performance were examined in 26,760 4-year-old American children who were born in the years 1959 through 1965. It was concluded that perinatal circumstances made a minor contribution to outcome as compared with the major effect of social factors. Low socioeconomic status of the family (as measured by educational attainment and occupation of the head of household, and by family income) was associated with a relatively high frequency of retarded development in the preschool children. The findings of these two large-scale studies were consistent with the conclusions in two smaller surveys reported in 1967 and 1970; again, social class variables had a much greater effect on intellectual development than did the presence of perinatal complications.

The outcome of the smallest and most immature infants cared for in neonatal intensive care units since 1970 (which roughly marks the beginning of the "modern technologic era") has been watched with much apprehension. It was important to know whether a fall in mortality among these babies could be achieved without paying a high price in terms of handicapped survivors. Drillien reported that between two 5-year periods (1948– 1952 incl. and 1955–1960), the survival rate of Edinburgh babies with birthweights of 1.36 kg (3 lb) or less had increased from 17 to 30 percent; the change was attributed to advances in perinatal care over the span of 12 years. Unfortunately, the increase in the survival rate seemed to have taken place at the cost of an increase in the proportion of moderately or severely damaged children among the survivors: the handicapped rate rose from 32 percent in 1948–1952 to 56 percent in 1955–1960. It was gloomily predicted that as the survival rate of infants of very low birthweight improved with the introduction of new life-saving methods, an increasing number of damaged children would survive. A series of reports from University College Hospital, London, set out to refute this disturbing assumption. Improved survival depends on the anticipation of biochemical and other abnormalities which the smallest infants are unable to withstand, it was noted. These abnormalities—such as oxygen-lack, low blood glucose, and elevated concentrations of the toxic yellow pigment, bilirubin—are all capable of damaging the brain, the English observers argued, and their prevention should lead to an improved outlook for mental development among the survivors. With these thoughts in mind, they reported (1971) the developmental progress of a group of infants who weighed 1.5 kg (3 lb 4 oz) or less at birth and who had been treated more vigorously than in the past and with the newly developed techniques. The survey suggested that the outlook had improved: among 72 surviving infants only 5 were abnormal and 4 were classified as "doubtful" (when examined at ages ranging from 9 months to 4¼ years). Further reports from the London group have argued that there is continuing improvement in the prognosis for the infants in the smallest and most immature ranks. And, the favorable outlook has been attributed to intensive methods of care. Several follow-up observations from other neonatal intensive care units have also presented encouraging accounts, although many of the children were still very young at the time of the reports.

An ongoing survey of the eye changes among infants in an intensive care nursery in Vancouver, British Columbia, was begun in January 1968 by McCormick. Between the years 1968 and 1976, he examined 2031 infants and he noted a sharp rise in the numbers of eye-damaged infants beginning in 1974. This increase was associated with a general increase in the number of infants admitted to the Canadian special care unit, with a considerable increase in the number of small infants transported from hospitals not equipped to care for sick newborn infants, and with an apparent rise in the survival rate of the smallest premature infants.

The interpretation of wholly descriptive surveys in medicine is difficult. The information has been particularly slippery in the perinatal field of inquiry because of the "built-in" problem of population selection and the practical difficulties of accounting for the effects of events which occur in the long interval between discharge from the hospital and the time of formal evaluation of the outcome. And, the interpretive difficulties have mounted in recent years. The demographic composition of the population of infants born alive, as I indicated earlier, has been changing rapidly. The development of regional programs for perinatal care has resulted in an increasing distortion in the selection of the population of infants in intensive care units (for example, one-half of the children in the original University College Hospital follow-up survey had been born in other institutions and were transferred to the specialized unit for care). In addition to these issues which raise problems in interpretation, there are questions introduced by changing policies in the vigor with which life-support measures are applied to infants who are severely compromised (e.g., severe malformations, prolonged asphyxia, suspected hemorrhage into the brain). To emphasize once more, there are unavoidable (but major) problems associated with the long interval which must elapse between the events in the perinatal period and the time when a reliable assessment of outcome can be made. In addition, the social environment in which children are reared has changed rapidly over time. Despite all of these difficulties in interpreting the practical effects of the new childbirth technology, surprisingly few doubts have been expressed concerning the favorable claims which have been made. I do not wish to imply that the rescue efforts have been fruitless, but what is missing is some *quantification* (from formal tests of specific interventions and an accounting of the multivariate influences which affect outcome). Difficult as it is to apportion the effects of the numerous changes which have been occurring, it seems mindless to ignore the complexity of the situation. And, in the face of the uncertainties, I believe it is unconscionable to lobby for increased investment in efforts focused on technologic escalations. The point is that the relation between outlay and outcome cannot be settled by the *ex post facto* evidence presently available. Furthermore, there is now a healthy skepticism about the cost-effectiveness of medical programs. Questions can no longer be put off by the kind of simplistic cause-and-effect assurances which sufficed in the past.

I indicated above that there is some evidence which suggests that the importance of perinatal events is small in comparison with the effects of socioeconomic circumstances during the first few years of child development. Sameroff and Chandler conducted a critical review of the available evidence on this subject. They pointed out that almost all perinatal follow-up studies have proceeded on the assumption that the developmental course of the human infant is a linear chain of efficient causes and invariant effects; particular characteristics of either the child or his parents should, therefore, predict the ultimate course of growth and development. And failure to predict later pathology has been taken as a mandate to initiate a new search for the elusive cause. On the other hand, an alternative developmental model regards the process of human evolvement as a more circuitous one, in which linear chains of causality are rare. According to the latter interpretation (the organismic model), children and their environments are undergoing regular restructuring: early perinatal factors that have enduring consequences are assumed to do so because of persistent influences acting throughout the life-span. This explication suggests that acute events in the perinatal period should have minimal long-term effects. It is assumed that "self-righting" influences are powerful forces which are disposed to the promotion of normal human development; protracted developmental disorders are found only in the presence of equally distorting influences. From this point of view, predictive failures in the study of developmental disorders are not attributable to missing links or other simple constructions. Instead, the defects are assumed to be related to inadequate knowledge regarding the complex of *mutual* influences that operate between the child and his environment. Together, these serve to dissipate or to amplify the effects of earlier developmental insults. To gain predictive validity from the perinatal influences one must take into account the maintaining environment. Sameroff and Chandler introduced the phrase "continuum of caretaking casualty" to characterize the circumstance which may arise when a disadvantaged family with poor emotional, physical, and economic resources must cope suddenly with the consequences of the birth of a premature or asphyxiated infant. This crisis is likely to put a burden on the parents' limited caretaking abilities. The chance that such a child will receive close and attentive care is further jeopardized by *his* influence on family interaction. The infant's disturbance in alertness, vigor, sucking, or stability of sleep/wake cycles has a cumulative and disrupting effect on the development of a smooth child–parent relationship. And, there is evidence to make the thesis of the "continuum of caretaking casualty" a fairly reasonable one. Neurologic signs present at 1 year of age in infants who are asphyxiated at birth tend to persist in children who grow up in disadvantaged environments. The outlook for infants (with similar birth histories and abnormal signs at 1 year) appears to be different if they are reared in socially advantaged settings: in many of these fortunate children, the signs disappear and many function normally by the age of 10 years. Werner and her associates analyzed the outcome of 1000 live births and concluded that perinatal complications were related to later physical and psychological development only when combined with and supported by persistently poor environmental circumstances. Moreover, the biologically vulnerable children constituted only a small proportion of the number who were not functioning normally at age ten. Ten times more children had problems related to the effects of poor early environment than to the effects of perinatal stress.

The studies cited by Sameroff and Chandler suffer from the same maddening shortcomings to which I have alluded. Nonetheless, there is at least as much evidence to support their interpretations as there is for the arguments concerning the singular effects of perinatal events. It would be shortsighted, Baum has recently noted, to ignore the influences of the child's environment on his development after a complicated course in the newborn period. I do not wish to exaggerate more than is necessary for effect, but to the extent that resources and efforts are focused exclusively on technologic support in pregnancy and delivery, I must say that planning vision is disturbingly limited. Doctor Laura Nader was moved to comment on the current situation at the conclusion of a conference in 1975 entitled "Critical Issues in Neonatal Intensive Care." Questions should be raised, she noted, about who benefits economically from neonatal intensive care: the companies that produce the life-support machinery, the doctors who work at this labor, insurance companies, the hospital, the parents, the families of the newborn infant, the baby? How has our society come to be spending so much time and money on neonatal intensive care, she asked, without similar attention to born healthy but later not-so-healthy, deprived children? These provocative questions remain unanswered.

12

Progress in a Groove

Perinatal medicine has sprouted and grown rapidly in the past 25 years. The same period has been marked by a gradual (and overall) erosion in public trust of the medical profession and its institutions. I do not wish to imply that there is a simple cause-and-effect relationship between these two developments, but I find it hard to ignore the fact that the new field of medical activity has been singled out for special criticism by community groups in the United States and in Great Britain. I believe, therefore, that it may be useful to attempt to trace the roots of community versus profession conflict. The areas I will explore in this chapter are the narrowness of outlook which results from the atomistic approach to complex problems, the demographic and social consequences of medical actions, clash of values, and a communication gap between community and profession.

Modern attempts to acquire a mechanistic understanding of outstanding medical problems (in terms of physiology and biochemistry) have taken the only route possible: the path of reductionism. A complex system must be broken down into manageable segments, and the isolated parts examined in depth. Nonetheless, the dissection approach to problem-solving is the beginning, not the end, of a search for solutions. The dangers of the present-day situation were recognized many years ago by Whitehead:

. . .a great fact confronting the modern world is the discovery of the method
of training professionals, who specialize in particular regions of thought and thereby add to the sum of knowledge within their respective limitations of subject . . .
this situation has its dangers. It produces minds in a groove. Each profession makes
progress, but it is progress in its own groove . . . Thus, in the modern world, the
celibacy of the medieval learned class has been replaced by the celibacy of the
intellect which is divorced from the concrete contemplation of the complete facts
. . . The dangers arising from this aspect of professionalism are great, particularly
in our democratic societies. The directive force of reason is weakened . . . In short,
the specialized functions of the community are performed better and more progressively, but the generalized direction lacks vision. The progressiveness in detail only
adds to the danger produced by the feebleness of coordination . . .

I believe that much of the public apprehension about modern perinatal
medicine has come about as a result of uncoordinated advance "in detail."
As the intensity of activities has increased, what seems to have been
ignored is that human infants are complex natural systems—they are wholes
with irreducible parts. Errors, misconceptions and disharmonies have crept
in as the focus of medical interest has narrowed to isolated biologic effects
(unrelated to the interconnected physico-chemical "systems" of the infant
organism) or to infants viewed out of context (as disconnected from inter-
grated social "systems" of the family, cultural group and community).

The profession should not be blamed for failing to foresee the unknown pathologic effect of supplemental oxygen on immature retinal blood
vessels. But, it must be criticized, I believe, for its failure to expect the
unexpected in the face of limitations of knowledge—to look beyond the
immediate outcome of interest (breathing pattern). And, this dereliction
occurred over and over with changes in feeding practices, administration of
new drugs, expansion of facilities, and proliferation of equipment. The
dangers of a narrow outlook are not confined to this field of medicine, but
the lessons are particularly revealing because the hazards are exaggerated
in the case of the fetus and newborn. In a figurative sense, these unknowing
patients have served a function which is like that provided by a miner's
canary: they have given early warning of the danger of increasing hazards
in medicine. The immature baby is a unique "species" of human being; he
exhibits an unusual vulnerability to minor changes in the chemical and
physical environment. For example, even the simple act of removing the
clothes of a premature infant in a warm-air, transparent incubator had a
major unexpected consequence. The focus of interest on observations of
the baby's respirations distracted attention away from the effect on heat
balance: there was a net loss of body heat through radiant exchange be-

tween the warm naked skin surface and the relatively cool Plexiglass walls of the incubator. The importance of this subtle physical effect was completely overlooked for years. Persistently low body temperature, under conditions of warm incubator-air temperature, was considered to be a "characteristic of prematurity" (newborn infants, unlike older individuals, do not shiver when body heat is lost). Finally, in 1958, a formal trial was conducted which demonstrated that during the first days of life, surprisingly small differences in body temperature were associated with vital effects: small newborn babies survived in increased numbers when heat dissipation via the radiant route of heat loss was compensated by increased warmth to bring body temperature up. These results were confirmed and, since the 1960s, an enormous amount of information has been collected concerning temperature regulation in the period immediately after birth. Many other perinatal phenomena are now reasonably well understood, but, compared to the pond of knowledge, our ignorance remains Atlantic. Ironically, it is the confidence in a firm foundation of evidence in isolated biologic effects which tends to encourage the daring jump to widespread everyday applications. All of the time and effort involved in working out the details of specific physiologic mechanisms under carefully regulated conditions make the slow (and, by contrast, crude) steps of formal evaluation at the bedside seem like annoying roadblocks which have been put up to retard progress. And, as therapeutic exuberance has increased, the dangers arising from the tunnel vision of the impatient specialist are greater now than ever.

In addition to effects on infants as individuals, there are some demographic consequences of perinatal actions which are of public concern. In the United States, the most common conditions associated with infant deaths are prematurity (and its complications) and congenital malformations. After the age of 40, heart disease, malignancies, and strokes account for more than half of all deaths. Efforts to prolong life in these two periods (before and after the years of procreation) produce population impacts which are quite unequal. The reverberations of actions taken in nurseries are greater by far than those taken in adult sections of hospitals. The asymmetry has been true in the past and the preeminent importance to the community of the outcomes of pregnancy will undoubtedly persist. The demographic effects are both quantitative and qualitative.

The steady increase in life expectancy in the United States since the beginning of this century has been due primarily to the fall in mortality rates during early infancy and childhood. Since 1900, the expected duration of life for an infant has increased by approximately 22 years, while the life expectancy for an American of 40 has lengthened by only 6 years.

Infant mortality in 1976 (15.1 deaths under 1 year of age per 1000 live births in the U.S.) was less than one-sixth of the rate 60 years earlier, and the decline in that year alone was the largest proportional drop in 20 years. Three-quarters of the deaths under 1 year take place in the first month after birth, and half of the infant deaths occur in the first 24 hours following delivery. Even small changes in the mortality rates at these early ages are reflected in large effects on present-day age distributions and on population size, and the effects are magnified in future generations: the rate of numerical increase in population is determined primarily by the numbers of children who reach the childbearing ages. Prolongation of life after the reproductive years has a relatively small and, of course, short term effect on total numbers of the population.

It is the survival of girls which tends to dominate effects on reproductive pressures and, thus, future population size. Harris has pointed out that this "explains" the frequent use of female infanticide as a population control measure in primitive societies who have no other means to balance the number of mouths to feed and the means of subsistence. For example, the number of births "expected" in a group of ten men and ten women would be the same as in a group consisting of one man and ten women. But, in a local group of ten men and only one woman, the birth rate "expected" would be one-tenth of the two other examples. All other things being equal, it is the number of women which determines the rate of reproduction. The sex composition of a population depends largely on the sex ratio among live born infants and the relative sex-specific mortality rates. As a result, it is of some interest to note that there are substantial differentials in the mortality of the sexes in infancy, particularly in the newborn period. More male infants are born (1054 males per 1000 females in the U.S. in 1975) but the disparity in numbers is quickly eroded by a striking excess of male mortality rates: the risk-margin in favor of girls is greatest in the first days and months; by 9–11 months of age the excess mortality among males narrows to 11 percent (Fig. 12-1). Mortality-risk for boys is greater than for girls at most birth weights (Fig. 12-2). The point to be made here is that the effect of reduction in early deaths (especially of small babies) is one of augmenting the ratio of females over males in the population. [For example, as infant mortality in the United States fell from the years 1940 to 1970, the percent excess of male over female mortality rates increased progressively (Table 12-1)]. A complex of effects may be felt in future generations, I suggest, as the result of present declines in birth rate and in perinatal mortality; age composition, sex ratio, and population size can be expected to be altered. My view of the potential

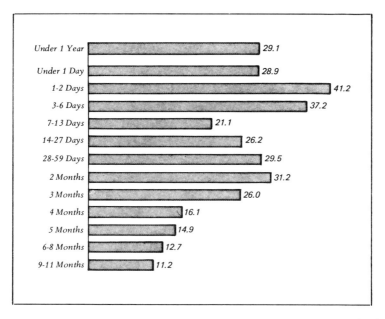

Fig. 12-1.   Percent excess of male over female mortality rates by age in the
United States (1959– 1961).

effects of current medical activities (although the exact contributions of
many specific actions have not been demonstrated, see p 94) differs from
McKeown's conclusion concerning influences in the past. He found that
medical measures have had relatively little effect on historical trends. The
exponential rise of world population since the 18th century can be accounted
for, in large part, by a fall in infant mortality. A main restraint on population growth before this time, McKeown observed, was the high level of
deaths brought about by the limited capacity of the environment (particularly the availability of food) to support the number of babies born. He
collected evidence which indicated that medical conquest of disease played
a minor role in the modern rise of population, and that the level of fertility
remained unchanged over this period. Obviously, the situation is changing
dramatically. As environmental limiting effects decline and technical control of fertility and of perinatal mortality become more efficient, the levers
which manipulate population numbers are (for the first time, if McKeown's
reading of history is correct) passing into medical hands.

The qualitative changes in demography resulting from intensified perinatal actions are difficult to measure. But information about genetic disor-

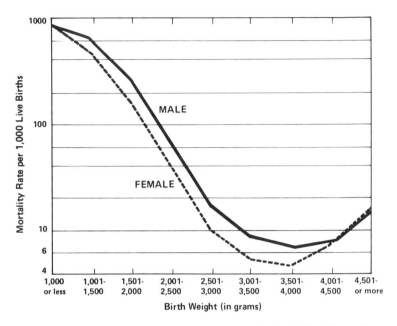

Fig. 12-2.   Mortality by birthweight in the two sexes in the United States (Jan.–Mar., 1950). Deaths under 28 days of age.

ders gives some clue about biologic changes which may be expected as perinatal mortality falls. For example, about 40 percent of conceptions end in spontaneous miscarriage; a little more than half of these occur so early that a woman may not know that she is pregnant. Major chromosomal abnormalities are a leading cause of this substantial toll of fetal life. Serious genetic defects are present in about 4 percent of all live-born infants; the rate increases progressively with decreasing maturity and birth weight (the proportion is particularly high in infants who are undergrown, i.e., birth weight lower than expected for duration of pregnancy). Malformations are also a leading cause of death in the first days after birth and in infancy. Erbe notes that birth defects claim as many "life years" as does heart disease, eight times as many as cancer, and ten times as many as stroke. Thus, even a minor change in the survival of fetuses and infants with birth defects has a major demographic impact. In 1977, it was estimated that 12 million Americans have genetically caused birth defects. About 20–30 percent of all hospital admissions of children are related primarily to genetic disorders, and it is estimated that malformations are

Table 12-1

Infant Mortality and Percent Excess of Male Mortality Rates
By Years (United States 1940– 1970)

Year*	All Infants	Males	Females	Percent Excess of Male Mortality
1940	47.0†	52.5†	41.3†	27.1
1950	29.2	32.8	25.5	28.6
1960	26.0	29.3	22.6	29.6
1970	20.4	23.3	17.5	33.1

*Live-birth sex ratio remained unchanged over this period: 1055 males per 1000 female live-births in 1940, exactly the same ratio in 1970.
†Deaths under 1 year of age per 1000 live births.

the commonest cause for hospitalization of children in North America. The net effect on these statistics of genetic screening programs during pregnancy, therapeutic abortion for identified genetic disorders, and falling perinatal mortality rates has not been calculated. And again, one can only guess about the effect projected to future generations which will result from the prolongation of life of children with serious heritable abnormalities. Consider, for example, the puzzles which are involved in cystic fibrosis. It is the most common, serious, recessively inherited disorder in the white population of the United States: it occurs in about one in 2000 births. The abnormality cannot, as yet, be diagnosed prenatally, and carriers (about 1/20 of the white population) cannot be identified. In the past, cystic fibrosis was considered to be uniformly fatal in infancy, many affected infants died soon after birth (often as the result of meconium ileus). Improvements in treatment have resulted in a steady increase in life-expectancy; the average age of survival was 15 years in 1970 and is now probably higher. From the community's point of view, the costs and benefits of medical efforts in cystic fibrosis can be computed by using relatively uncomplicated economic weightings. But the biologic issues involved in working through the full consequences of medical policies for meconium ileus (and in other severe genetic disorders which are evident at birth) are enormously complex. And they cannot be dismissed by the phrase "of academic interest only."

I do not find it surprising that the difficult dilemmas posed by developments in perinatal medicine have been greeted with widespread apprehension in this country. Moreover, it is concern about drawing the line in the rescue efforts which has acted as a wedge in widening the gap of disagreement between the community and the medical profession. Chargaff has pointed to an unfortunate tendency which he associates with the current revulsion from science: we have begun to believe that the fact that something can be done carries its own justification. He terms this the "devil's doctrine": what can be done must be done. As noted above, the disharmony is not confined to the United States. In 1974, for example, a consumer group in England found more adverse comments about maternity services than any other branch of medical practice. Chalmers noted with interest that this criticism surfaced in Oxford, a city which had attained one of the lowest perinatal mortality rates in the United Kingdom. Even in developing countries with high rates of perinatal loss, the new childbirth technology has received a mixed reception. Medical staffs of health ministries strive to improve coverage of overall health services, rather than investment in expensive technology which benefits relatively few patients. But administrators lack the charisma of intensive-care specialists. The voice of caution has often gone unheeded. However, there is some evidence of general disillusion with high-cost, high-technology medicine which operates only within a relatively sophisticated environment. In many countries, the value of intensive technologic approaches has been seriously questioned when measured in terms of their impact on improving the health status of the populations. An article in the Bangladesh Times (Jan. 14, 1977) is revealing. The commentator called attention to an example of advice from western consultants which was completely unrealistic for his people and the environment: a laparoscope was recommended for every rural health center in Bangladesh. This highly sensitive, sophisticated instrument requires both electricity and gas to function; not all hospitals in Britain have a laparoscope, the reporter exclaimed. The same article also told of a discussion between the reporter and a friend from abroad. The visitor said that he had encountered 72 foreign advisors in Dacca on that day alone. "And yourself?", the writer asked. "Seventy-three," was the admission. The newsman concluded that it will be an uphill road, overcoming this favorable bias toward the wisdom of the west. Such an effort was made in 1974 at a workshop arranged by the West African Health Secretariat and convened in Ghana. The members of the workshop from five African nations recommended that highly trained doctors will have to consider accepting constraints on some activities hitherto regarded as sacrosanct. Lewis Mumford came to a similar conclusion in another, not entirely dissimilar, context. In 1946 he reviewed the crisis brought on by the advent of the nuclear age; he outlined a program for survival and pleaded that we do not forget the most essential secret of humankind's advance; the practice of restraint.

What are the social effects of medical efforts to rescue fetuses and newborn infants? As I have indicated, the operations are more than technical achievements to be measured by vital statistics. They are social actions with powerful long-term effects on individuals. And, it is in the consequences of technical actions as seen in persons—taken one by one—that the "danger produced by the feebleness of coordination" is particularly high. The experience with RLF is illustrative of the failed opportunities to go beyond the limitations of an organ-bound perspective. For example, the huge 1953–54 Cooperative Study of RLF (as a condition affecting the eye) was disbanded after a year. But, the full expression of the chronic condition know as RLF-blindness (affecting the whole child, the family, social agencies, schools and community) was just beginning. In the past few years, I have contacted RLF-blinded young adults and, later, some of the parents to ask about their life experiences. I was surprised to learn that the young men and women (in their twenties) had only vague information about RLF and theories about the mechanism of the oxygen effect. Very few knew any details of the epidemic or about the national efforts to study the disorder and to control the outbreak. Many told me they had been puzzled for years; their parents and physicians seemed restrained by what the young people felt was a conspiracy of silence about the entire subject. I organized several small groups for informal marathon discussions. I told them everything I knew about the history and the medical aspects of the disorder; they told me what it was like to grow up without vision in the United States. I learned very quickly that loss of sight is not the major burden faced by blind children and young adults. Preconceptions, paternalism and insensitivity of authorities in the visually oriented world constrict the lives of those who wish to see this same world nonvisually.

Discussions with parents, singly and in groups, were much more difficult for me (and for them). Most of the parents were still bitterly angry at the medical profession, but not for the reason I imagined. They understood and accepted the fact of limited knowledge at the time their children were born. Most were convinced that physicians had rendered excellent care and had used supplemental oxygen liberally in well-meant efforts to improve the chances of the small babies for intact survival. But, almost without exception, parents recalled (with rancor) that once the diagnosis of RLF was made, a chill in relationships developed. At the very time when they needed support and advice, their physicians became distant and defensive, the parents recalled. Most blamed their doctors for failing to maintain interest and concern, not for the failure of clairvoyance! The parents said it was anger at personal, not professional, behavior of physicians, which prompted many of the RLF legal suits charging malpractice which burgeoned in this country.

There is no accurate method of estimating the total number of malpractice law suits, alleging improper use of oxygen, which have been initiated since the 1950s. Some of the actions have been launched when the affected are in their twenties. (This is made possible by the fact that the statute of limitations is reckoned from the time of attaining the legal age of majority; the periods vary from state to state.) There are no satisfactory national statistics which total the decisions reached in legal actions; some have been settled out of court, others have been tried and the opinions are unreported. Several leaders in the blind community have told me that one must not minimize the disservice to the blind which has resulted from these law suits and the publicity announcing enormous awards of money. The actions run counter to the course of the changing status of the blind in our society. There is a move from dependence toward independence and the young adults are ready to demonstrate that their visual loss need not be handicapping if they are given an opportunity to demonstrate their competence. The huge sympathy awards perpetuate the tin-cup stereotype which they wish to erase. If a fraction of the time and money spent in legal battles over RLF were channeled into efforts to provide meaningful employment for blind young hopefuls (physicians and lawyers should be leading the way) our national guilt would be harnessed effectively. Most parents are bitter about the unfair barriers to employment which are being encountered by their children.

I found the discussions with parents extremely disturbing. The problems associated with visual disability seemed minor compared to the endless struggles with members of the helping professions, teachers, and schools (parents fought for years and finally were successful—because of the large numbers of RLF-blinded children—in bringing about a shift in school placement from segregation in residential schools to integration with sighted schoolmates). I was acutely aware of the fact that these interviews with a selected group of parents who had coped successfully could never provide an accurate picture of the full range and incidence of social problems (e.g., abandonment, child abuse, divorce, suicide) associated with the largest oubreak of blindness in American history. The opportunity to obtain reliable information (which would have been useful in developing social support for affected families) was missed in the 1950s.

I do not wish to give the impression that it would have been a simple matter to mount a multidisciplined, long-term study of this complex disorder (which I now envision with the wisdom of hindsight). I must emphasize, however, that this was an early example of the disparity between community need and the pattern of clinical investigation. A high-priority question for the community was, What are the social consequences of RLF-blindness? But, it was a low-priority question for medical inquiry (and the question was never addressed in a systematic fashion). This kind of divergence (not exclusive to medicine) provoked a perceptive editorial by Commoner under the heading "The Responsibility of Science." He suggested that the disparities arise in a number of ways, some of which have little to do with intellectual challenge (popularly viewed as the motivational stimulus for research). There is a tendency to shun slow-paced, but socially important, studies, he noted, given the present criteria for accomplishment in science: economic support and academic acclaim depend on a high volume of production of publications. His point must not be ignored in debates about the level of public funding for medical studies. I believe that the disincentives of the reward system in clinical research (particularly economic pressure for quick results) did play a role in discouraging organized study of the social consequences of RLF. And it goes a long way in explaining why information concerning the social costs of perinatal rescue operations is so incomplete: studies have focused on the outcome status of individuals—survival, neurologic and intellectual status—rather than the outcome in families and communities. A recent prospective study in North Carolina indicates a disturbingly high rate of social chaos in the families of infants discharged from a newborn intensive care unit (the risk of abuse and neglect was eight times higher than the "expected" rate in the state). The need for more long-term sociologic study is obvious.

While many problems which I have reviewed can be blamed on lack of foresight, technical limitations, or ignorance, there also were other unconscionable failures related to "the feebleness of coordination." For example, with the help of a superb team of technical experts at Babies Hospital, I once reared a premature infant who weighed 800 grams (1 lb 8 oz) at birth. Three months and several tens of thousands of dollars after birth, the infant was sent home to a Harlem flat. Within a week, we heard that the infant died at night when a rat chewed off his nose. This gruesome example of final results in what might be called the destructiveness of thoughtless benevolence recalls Tom Lehrer's bitter lyric about rocket weaponry:

Once they're up, who cares where they come down, That's not my department, says Wernher von Braun.

Repugnant as it is to say so, this brutally immoral attitude does shed light on an important dichotomy. Unlike the physician with a rescue fantasy, the weaponry specialist makes a clear distinction between technical decisions and value decisions. Brody observed that scientists or clinicians are prone to confuse scientific problems with value problems and try to solve the latter with tools of the former. But what is the role of professional knowledge in human affairs? In a number of ways, Freidson has suggested, medicine offers the best test of the general question of whether the ends of established professions are so beneficent that experts may be given the autonomy to lead all of society to them. In medicine, actions are based on reliable objective evidence and what the profession deems to be good, the public, on the surface, regards as good. However, there lies at the bottom of medicine's applied efforts, he correctly observes, a moral, rather than an objective, stance. Further, the professionally defined "good" is asserted to be worth the price the patient is asked to pay in relinquishing his independence. But, unless the moral foundation of medicine is identical to that of the community, Freidson concludes, it will serve not the community but itself.

Earlier, I argued that physicians should closely examine the biologic and social consequences of their actions. However, I must emphasize that it is not suggested that increased sensitivity justifies dominance in the realm of values. The role of a perceptive and sympathetic consultant should not be confused with that of a moral arbiter or an agent of social control. A WHO study group has affirmed the information-giving role of physicians (as opposed to a controlling function) when difficult ethical problems arise in the management of newborn infants with multiple congenital defects. They advised that, as a general rule, decisions should be those of the parents. The physician should be concerned with explaining to the parents, as accurately as possible, the consequences of available options, the group urged. Freidson examined the limits of professional authority, and concluded that the professions, no matter how beneficent their intent, have neither the moral right nor the special qualifications to make choices for the individual or for society. Physicians often make the assumption that "Medical Practice" (especially when it is based on scientifically sound principles) is a pure, moral, acultural phenomenon. I believe that it is this issue—the conflict between the value judgments of doctors and individual families—which has been a major difficulty in the development of perinatal medicine. The clash was discussed at a conference entitled, "Values Underlying the New Childbirth Technology" in 1977. Participants from a number of disciplines (including child development, economics, history, midwifery, obstetrics, pediatrics, philosophy and policy planning) uncovered many deviations in outlook based on the degree to which pregnancy and childbirth were seen primarily as medical events, or psychological and social events which occasionally require medical assistance. When parent and physician differ in pregnancy and childbirth, who should make decisions concerning care?, was one of the numerous questions debated. Peter Steinfels argued that childbirth, and pregnancy as well, have been transformed into a "medical model" and pregnant women have been assigned a "sick role." This modern shift has a number of debatable consequences: it mobilizes the coercive power of labels (the terms "low risk" and "high risk" have become judgmental, like "good" and "bad," "legal" and "illegal"); it shifts authority to the physician and the setting to the hospital; it casts the pregnant patient in a passive role and minimizes her sense of responsibility; and, finally, it justifies the use of specialized, technical, and often very expensive approaches and treatments. As a result, he noted, the childbirth experience has been isolated from other realms of meaning. It has become primarily a medical event rather than a family event, a religious event, or a special moment in the life cycle. This cogent analysis met with vigorous opposition from the medical conferees who argued for a continuation of professional control. The debates served to underline the wide divergence of views among the learned disciplines and the genuine difference in fundamental values among Americans.

I suggest that as knowledge concerning the fetus and newborn has deepened, the profession has sallied forth from the laboratories carrying "truth" on a banner with the same missionary spirit which guided the New England clerics when they invaded Tikopia with Godly truth and stamped out the Melanesian population-control practice of infanticide. But, the frantic evangelism of modern perinatal medicine is puzzling. Given the dismal record of hasty, unevaluated actions in the past, one may very properly ask: What in God's name is the hurry? One possible answer is provided by historians who have reviewed the Puritan outlook on science and medicine. Webster detects an underlying millenarianism: an attempt to return to the pure state of Adam before the Fall, when man had insight into all truth and power over the created world; when this is achieved the millenium is to be at hand. The evangelist's drive and hurry to achieve the millenium should be obvious to anyone who looks at the record of the medical science effort of the past few decades. And the quasi-religious fervor has been characteristic of the growth of technology in general. Mumford notes that the demands of mechanical progress have had the effect of a divine ordinance, sacrilegious to challenge, impossible to disobey.

Medicine's imperative resembles that of fundamentalist religions; the similarity emerges when its value-system clashes with other fundamentalist groups. The Jehovah's Witness faith, for example, interprets biblical passages from Genesis ("Only flesh with its soul—its blood—you must not eat.") and from Leviticus (". . . the soul of every sort of flesh is its blood. Anyone eating it will be cut off.") as a proscription against blood transfusions. When parents of a newborn infant refuse to consent to an exchange blood transfusion on the grounds of religious freedom, doctors have appealed (successfully) to the courts for permission. This dilemma is usually argued in terms of the limits of the rights of parenthood, but, I suggest, it points up the issue of conflicting value judgements. And, it poses questions concerning the limits of the rights of the dominant culture in a plural society to impose its values on a minority. Brody notes that ethics involves choosing among options which are probability estimates on possible future states, by a process of weighing them against a set of values. The Witnesses keep their eyes on the future prize of everlasting life and they choose not to evoke God's wrath by breaking His law to extend their lives for only a temporary period of time through blood transfusions. Their children, whose lives have been prolonged ("saved" is a term used in medical fundamentalism) by exchange transfusion, grow up with the belief that they alone, among their co-religionists, have been denied eternal life. These unhappy results of medicine's self-righteousness recall one of George Bernard Shaw's maxims for revolutionists, "Do not do unto others as you would that they should do unto you. Their tastes may not be the same."

The problem of whether moral principles are absolute or relative is an ancient theme in ethics. As I reflect on the dismal results of the moral stands about which I once felt so certain, I find myself siding with those who argue that there is no ethical principle that is acknowledged by all human societies. And I am more willing than ever to accept the view that morals are socially agreed upon values relating to conduct. To this extent morals (and all group values) are the products of social interaction as embodied in culture. These interpretations emphasize that an individual's or group's conceptions of what is and what ought to be are intimately connected. And, it follows that the evaluation of risk versus benefit in all medical interventions, proven and experimental, is a highly difficult and individualized process in a multicultural society like the United States.

It has been particularly hard to make value judgments concerning experiments involving human beings. For example, Beecher, in 1966, described 50 clinical studies which he believed violated ethical standards. He arbitrarily selected the intent of the experimenter as the axis of categorization, not the observed risk. This approach has been widely accepted in the past decade. Beecher's classes have been summarized into two mutually exclusive categories: "therapeutic" and "nontherapeutic" research. But does it fit the real world in which the line between "therapy" and "nontherapy" can rarely be drawn? In addition to philosophic vagaries, placebo–reactor effects blur such neat categorizations. And, more disturbing, this blurring gives rise to deliberate evasions when "nontherapeutic" research is proscribed. Beecher's dichotomous view of the world of clinical studies is held by many physicians. It is a hold-over from medicine's past which was ruled by authoritative judgments rather than critical rationalism. The two-value orientation clashes with the scientific view of the world which is probabilistic: judgments are tentative and based on a shifting body of evidence; classifications tend to be scalar rather than categorical. In my opinion, medicine is in the midst of an identity crisis, as it struggles to become scientific. And, I believe, the ambiguity has much to do with the Babel-like atmosphere prevailing in various public forums which have been convened in recent years to discuss the subject of experimentation involving helpless subjects.

Medicine's slow and uneven shift from mystical certainty to scientific uncertainty has led to a gap in communication between the profession and the community. I suspect there is a feeling of betrayal and confusion at this turn of events. Doctors are viewed suspiciously when they ask questions—a switch from their accustomed role as providers of answers. For example, the Vivisection Investigation League sent out a flier damning controlled experiments on the effects of temperature in premature infants (Fig. 12-3). The writer of the brochure completely misunderstood the question which was addressed by the study and his statements were misleading. In fact, the temperature trial compared survival among infants reared under the standard warming method (used in this country for many years) with the outcome under a new method which kept infants *warmer*. Survival in the first days of life was improved under the new conditions. Moreover, the question Should newborn babies be kept warm?, turned out to be more complicated than it appeared to the League. Subsequent studies demonstrated that the advantage was temporary. When the warmer conditions were maintained for more than a week, the babies had decreased cold resistance; if inadvertently exposed to the cold during bathing or feeding, they had a diminished capacity to prevent a fall in body temperature.

Public unease with a medical profession that asks questions has also been reflected in the relationships with legislators. One example may illustrate the disturbing consequences of the climate of mistrust. In 1967, a

Should New Born Babies Be Kept Warm?

From instinct animals know that it is well to keep a new born baby close to the mother's body for warmth. There was a time when, without consulting "scientists," babies were rubbed with oil after delivery, wrapped in blankets and put into bed with their mothers.

Then came the "scientific era." Babies were taken from their mothers, bathed and put into baskets in sterilized nurseries where the temperature was controlled. But it was still generally accepted that babies should be kept warm. Especially those that were born prematurely.

However, after repeated experiments on baby animals, exposing them to warm and cold environments, directly after birth, the scientific mind was intrigued. Did a neonate animal respond to its environment like an adult, and if so how did it adjust to changes in temperature?

And how about HUMAN babies? Just how would it be if they were NOT kept warm after birth? Would survival be greater or less in a warm environment?

Dr. Richard Day, Pediatrician, University of Pittsburgh made a "controlled" study of 125 babies weighing between 600 and 1,900 grams (or premature babies). In some babies Dr. Day carefully regulated the temperature, in others he did not.

In his first experiments with 125 babies, the warm babies had only 23% mortality while in the "control" group 37% died. (Note the term "control group" which is always used by experimenters when referring to the animals they use without treatment.)

Dr. Day REPEATED his experiments and again found that of the warm babies only 18% died, while in the "control" group the mortality was 49%.

(Perhaps mothers of the premature babies would have been glad if ALL the babies had been kept in a well regulated, warm environment.)

Send for Our New Brochure Before Your Prematurely Born Child
or Grandchild Falls Into the Hands of Experimenters...It DOES
HAPPEN even at So-Called First Class Hospitals!

Fig. 12-3. Flier circulated by Vivisection Investigation League – Antivivisection Society of New York in the 1960s.

118

New York State senator created headlines in New York City's tabloid, The Daily News, with a claim that inhuman experiments in children were being conducted in New York City Municipal Hospitals. He drafted legislation to outlaw all experimentation in children. Deans of medical schools in the state formed an ad hoc group to lobby against the proposed action. This group asked Doctors Joseph Dancis, Lawrence Finberg, and me to draft a white paper on the subject. We prepared a document which advised that the usual defensive posture of academic medicine should be abandoned in favor of a positive approach to deal with the real and unsolved problems. We noted that there was substance to the charge that clinical investigation was conducted more among the poor than among those on higher rungs of the socioeconomic ladder, and that informed consent for studies of the young and helpless was an unsolved problem. We proposed that there should be legislation in the form of an enabling law to encourage properly safeguarded clinical studies involving children, and that a permanent Commission be formed to work on the problem of finding acceptable solutions to the ongoing impediments to proper, scientifically rigorous studies in children.

The senator's threat was sufficiently grave to cause the president of the Society for Pediatric Research to devote his address to the subject of experimentation in children at the annual meeting of that group in the spring of 1967. The Society's leader concluded by announcing a Joint Committee on Clinical Investigation in Children which he would chair. Additional representatives from the American Pediatric Society, National Institute of Child Health and Human Development, National Association of Pediatric Department Chairmen and the American Academy of Pediatrics were appointed, I among them. But the committee never met! The senator dropped his attack and the proposed legislation the moment he lost the headlines. And we dropped our responsibility the minute the threat to business-as-usual was removed. Eight years later, I reviewed this episode with one of the principals, and we both agreed that we erred in following legal advice to "lay low." Subsequent events and the present-day situation indicate how wrong we were not to pursue this matter in a responsible way in 1967. We differed about a judgment concerning additional forces at work. I insisted that the threats to the flow of money for research were met with hasty efforts to sweep all of the untidy bits and pieces under the rug out of view.

The 1967 alarm had the effect of encouraging "bootleg" studies which fall somewhere between the kind of informal studies which I have described in Chapter 10 and formal planned trials. Disguised experiments are those in which research-oriented physicians consciously undertake a series of steps into the unknown without a formal plan or formal peer review. Arguing that bold new treatments are not experimental, but merely "modification or evolution of existing practice" and "based on sound physiologic principles," they proceed to treat a group of patients. Sticky issues of informed consent and strict review are simply side-stepped. The discipline of the scientific method is ignored in these trials. An example (and it is not unusual) is a study which began early in 1969. A newborn premature infant with severe respiratory distress was treated with a technique (continuous positive airway pressure) which had never been used before in newborn infants. The state of oxygenation in the blood of this infant improved; oxygen concentration in the inspired air was lowered and the seriously ill infant survived. Signed parental consent was not obtained for this new treatment. Contrary to the rules for experimentation involving human subjects which were circulated by the National Institutes of Health in 1966, signed permission was not obtained before the new treatment was applied to 19 more patients with severe respiratory distress. A formal protocol of study was not drawn up or reviewed by a Committee for Human Investigation. There were no randomly assigned concurrent controls who received the standard accepted treatment. Despite all of these violations of the letter and the spirit of the rules governing scientific human experimentation, the study was accepted for presentation at the annual meeting of the Society for Pediatric Research in 1970. Subsequently, the results were accepted for publication by reviewers and editors of the prestigious New England Journal of Medicine.

There have been surprisingly few objections to this kind of poor clinical science that led to the RLF epidemic and to the other catastrophes I have cataloged in Chapter 10. On the contrary, the "Russian roulette" strategy has been condoned and widely praised. Responsible efforts to conduct randomized clinical trials of proclaimed treatments have been characterized as "daring." One commentator wrote:

> While controlled trials are always comforting, it's probably not a very effective way to assess therapy which may be dependent on a number of variables.

As one attempts to summarize the disharmonies which have accompanied the unprecedented advances in biomedical knowledge in recent years, one point stands out: there is a rift in communications between the medical profession and the community. Physicians have one foot in the empirical past, the other in the new age of scientific inquiry. An ambivalent profession has failed to send out a clear message: early bedside applications are always a leap into the dark. The tedious approach of controls and replications used to reduce the risk of errors in preclinical investigations is needed even more at the clinical step where the complexity and heterogeneity of the interconnected "systems" increase abruptly. In the face of this increased uncertainty, the need for the cautious, hedging discipline of the scientific method increases correspondingly. In the United States there are conflicting attitudes and interests concerning the formats to be used in guiding the application of new knowledge, and all of the clashes are intensified if children are involved. Physicians, who should be in the forefront explaining the principles of the scientific method to parents, politicians, lawyers, etc., are themselves largely alienated from the discipline of planned clinical investigations. But the problem has been growing for some time. It was recognized by Claude Bernard more than 100 years ago when he wrote:

Many physicians attack experimentation on human beings believing that medicine should be a science of observation, but physicians make therapeutic experiments daily on their patients, so this inconsistency cannot stand careful thought. Medicine is by its nature an experimental science, but must apply the experimental method systematically.

13

The Experimental Method in Clinical Studies of Children

Lawyers and judges have denounced the Cooperative Study of RLF during some of the malpractice court trials in which I have testified. There is moral outrage because of the procedure of assigning infants to oxygen treatments by lot in the formal study which brought the epidemic to a swift end. But no word of criticism is expressed against the 12 years of informal experimentation in which physician-prescribed treatments led to the blinding of 10,000 children. The controlled trial of chloramphenicol, which ended the "gray syndrome" epidemic (p 82), was attacked in the United States Senate for the same reason (assignments by lot). The situation is bizarre. As I have shown earlier, a doctor may (with impunity) prescribe a "fashionable" untested treatment because of the advice of an authority or a colleague who is a personal friend; because he has read about it in the newspapers, in advertisements, or in medical journals; or simply because the treatment "makes good physiologic sense." On the other hand, if he should decide that there is sufficient uncertainty to warrant caution, and he chooses to undertake a planned test, his action is subject to criticism. "I need permission to give a new drug to half my patients, but not to give it to them all," said Smithells, commenting on the absurdity of this situation.

I agree with Smithells; it is difficult to understand this state of affairs.

It seems to have something to do with intent. If the physician causes death and maiming as the result of well-intentioned guessing, this is tolerated because it is not perceived as "experimentation." And theologically oriented bioethicists are firm about the decisive importance of "intention": expiation is sanctified by good intentions. However, from the patient's point of view, this semantic myopia is hardly comforting. The uninterpretable results of crude trial-and-error studies seem to be tolerated by society, but the patients are seldom heard from. I discussed the opposing strategem— formal experiment—with RLF-blinded young adults. They had no difficulty understanding the need for the controlled-trial approach in 1953–54 (including assignments by lot) given the dilemmas of that time.

In connection with drug experimentation and the public conscience, Edmund Cahn has commented on a pious fraud. He calls it the "Pompey Syndrome" (named for Sextus Pompey who appears in Shakespeare's *Anthony and Cleopatra*). Cahn relates:

Pompey, whose navy has won control of the seas around Italy, comes to negotiate peace with the Roman triumvirs . . . and they meet in a roistering party on Pompey's ship. As they carouse, one of Pompey's lieutenants draws him aside and whispers that he can become the lord of all the world if he will only grant the lieutenant leave to cut first the mooring cable and then the throats of the triumvirs. Pompey pauses, then replies in these words:

> "Ah, this thou shouldst have done,
> And not have spoke on't! In me tis
>   villany;
> In thee't had been good service.
>   Thou must know
> 'Tis not my profit that does
>   lead mine honour;
> Mine honour, it. Repent that
>   e'er thy tongue
> Hath so betrayed thine act; being
>   done unknown
> I should have found it afterwards
>   well done,
> But must condemn it now. Desist
>   and drink."

Cahn continues, very elegantly:

. . . here we have the most pervasive of moral syndromes, the one most characteristic of so called respectable man in civilized society. To possess the end and yet not be responsible for the means, to grasp the fruit while disavowing the tree, to escape being told the cost until someone else has paid it irrevocably; this is the "Pompey Syndrome" and the chief hypocrisy of our time. In the days of the outcry against thalidomide, how much of popular indignation might be attributed to this same syndrome; how many were furious because their own lack of scruple had been exposed?

The point is well taken. We cannot evade responsibility by shutting our eyes to the means used for gathering "intelligence" in medical warfare. Physicians, lawyers and judges are well versed on the subject of "evidence." No one in these professions can plead ignorance about the logical basis of the experimental method (or the special form of experimentation— the controlled trial—which has been available to contain the dimensions of treatment disasters). On the other hand, persons-on-the-street should not be accused of hypocrisy because the public has been so poorly informed about the risk-limiting alternatives to the primitive trial-and-error methods which are used so frequently to evaluate innovations. Accordingly, I would like to turn now to some of the ideas which underlie the experimental method and to some of the conflicts which account for resistance to this approach in studies involving children.

Informal, yet accurate, ongoing personal observations of the natural world have always been accepted as fundamental to progress; however, organized observations and enumeration were later refinements of the observational method of inquiry. Their introduction into medicine was slow and acceptance was uneven. Formal rules to guard against the problems of guessing and personal bias in arriving at conclusions in studies at the bedside have been developed only in the recent past. The format of the controlled clinical trial was perfected after World War II (within the "life-history" of the RLF incident).

The London Bills of Mortality, which date from 1603 onward, marked the beginning of the numerical approach to description of medical events. However, for many years the death rolls in parishes (and the fatalities of infants contributed disproportionately to the totals) were used merely to warn the Sovereign of the need to move into Clean Air. Greenwood reviewed the early period in the history of medical statistics, and in the papers and correspondence of a skeptical English physician, William Petty, he came upon some novel questions for the Bills to answer:

Whether of 1000 patients to the best physicians, aged of any decade, there do not die as many as out of the inhabitants of places where there dwell no physicians. Whether of 100 sick of acute diseases who use physicians, as many die and in misery, as where no art is used, or only chance.

Although these particular analyses were never carried out, the seed of the idea of formal comparisons was planted, and Greenwood suggests that out of the casual correspondence between Petty and his friend, John Graunt, in the mid-17th century, a new method of scientific investigation germinated and grew slowly. It is an irony of history that the idea developed more rapidly in other fields of biology than in medicine. Agricultural scientists, for example, took up the approach of systematic comparisons because of the practical difficulties in their work. They encountered the kind of problems found in medicine; different from those found in the physical sciences. For instance, physicists developed a method of observation and experiment which studied one factor at a time. To learn how pressure changes the volume of a gas, the temperature was kept constant. The physical experiment was limited, and isolated from its environment; but this kind of isolation was rarely possible in working with living things. Agricultural experimenters who wished to study the effects of fertilizers had to contend with innumerable and varying environmental influences. They could not eliminate them, yet their variations threatened to mask the singular effect of fertilizer. The techniques of numerical comparison of observations which I will discuss shortly, permitted the experimenters to work with evidence as they found it, and to measure an effect against the background of variation. They did not try to idealize an experiment, and instead accepted reality. The move from observations to a kind of experimentation which made it possible to approach the problem of uncontrollable confounding factors in a real-world setting was a major step in the biologic sciences.

The great French physiologist, Claude Bernard, proposed an operational approach to the acquisition of new information in medicine, by making a clear distinction between "observation" and "experiment." In his famous monograph, *An Introduction to the Study of Experimental Medicine* (1865), he noted that

In a philosophic sense, observation shows, and experiment teaches . . . in all experimental knowledge there are three phases: an observation made, a comparison established, and a judgment rendered.

He classified "observation" into two classes:

. . . A spontaneous or passive observation which the physician makes by chance and without being led to it by any preconceived idea . . . [secondly] an active observation . . . made with a preconceived idea, with intention to verify the accuracy of a mental conception.

The next step, "a comparison made", is the essence of the experimental method, but it has always been the most difficult to carry out in clinical medicine. The problems, well-exemplified in the history of the RLF epidemic, are of two principal kinds: psychologic difficulties and intellectual blocks.

The psychologic problems in experimental studies which involve children are generated by the nature of the interpersonal relationship between physician and parents. The authoritarian model bequeathed to medicine from the past assigns an all-knowing role to the physician. When the doctor confesses his uncertainty (the only stance possible in medical investigation), he threatens the very core of the relationship. It is pointless to argue about whose emotional needs are served by maintaining the fiction of physician omniscience, since both parties are thereby calmed. When a physician considers saying to a parent, "Your baby is going blind with RLF and I don't know how to prevent it," he comes face to face with his own need to grasp at straws in order to keep the authoritarian model afloat. Freidson examined this aspect of the professional role; he pointed out that client-oriented physicians (those who depend, primarily, on patients for approval) have more difficulty in unmasking than do their colleague-oriented coevals (those who depend on other physicians for approval). The subject deserves more careful study than it has received. The emotional entanglement of physician and parent has been a major factor in distracting both from the very real need of the infant patient for low-risk evaluation strategies in the contemporary world of powerful treatments, where the frightful consequences of guessing wrong have been magnified immeasurably.

The intellectual obstructions to the proper application of the experimental method in studies which involve children lie in the realm of statistics. There is widespread lack of understanding of the rationale of statistical techniques. This is the nub of a problem which seems to improve very little because of stubborn resistance, if not outright antipathy, to a revolutionary thought in modern science. Bronowski said of the statistical method, "It replaces the concept of *inevitable effect* by that of the *probable trend."*

Physicians have been reluctant to give up the idea of inevitable effect. Indeed, there is a long history of positivism in medicine which is difficult to overcome. The ideas of Galen (A.D. 138–201), which endured without challenge in the Western world for 16 centuries, typified the dogmatic approach. He codified a system of medicine based on his vast experience and on dissections of animals. The general approach was teleologic: Nature acts with perfect wisdom, he held, and from this credo he erected an authoritarian schema of diagnosis and treatment. A revealing aphorism ascribed to Galen reads:

> All who drink of this remedy recover in a short time, except those whom it does not help, who all die. Therefore, it is obvious that it fails only in incurable cases.

This type of positivist reasoning has persisted into the modern era. It played a role in delaying the solution to every medical problem I have described in this book. The view is reflected best in the 1953 report advising detergent-mist (". . . this is almost an infallible weapon . . .," p 74) and in the 1964 New York Times report of epsom-salt enemas ("It is not yet certain that the theory is correct, but it is certain that the treatment works," p 87). When we administered ACTH to infants with early RLF (p 22), were strongly tempted to explain away Galen-like) the "failures" of treatment. Even after we demonstrated that the initial impression of good results could not be substantiated by a comparative trial, some physicians continued to use this "remedy" because *their* results were good. Such dogged convictions based on personal experience have been a major stumbling block in modern medicine. They stand in the way of objective evaluation of new proposals once they have been applied widely. The attitudes are similar to those found in the South Pacific. At the time of a solar eclipse, islanders blow whistles, shout, and beat drums to frighten the moon into disgorging the sun. When this intervention is challenged, the "therapists" reply, in effect, "Why change, it works."

As I said earlier, statistical methodology (the probable trend approach) was taken up early by the biologic sciences because it provided a key to the puzzle of interpreting effects which tend to be obscured by variation. The central question in the studies of living things is how to decide whether an observed event is to be attributed to the meaningless play of chance on the one hand, or to causation or planned design on the other. There would be no need to invoke the logic of chance if we had to make inferences only about inevitable effects—nonvarying events. If *all* babies exposed to supplemental oxygen became blind, I would feel just as certain about one baby as I would about all infants so treated. Whatever the value of the generalization, it is neither greater or less than that of the particular statement: this baby exposed . . . became blind. The deductive process of inferring from the general to the particular in the class of nonvarying events, Venn taught 100 years ago, is not accompanied by the slightest diminution of certainty. He emphasized: if one of the "immediate inferences" is justified at all, it will be equally right in every case. But, unfortunately, this one-and-all characteristic applies to few events in the natural world, and it is rare (Galen-type declarations to the contrary notwithstanding) in medicine. The inferences we must make about medical events have a very different quality: as they increase in particularity, they diminish in certainty. Let me explain. Since *some* babies exposed to oxygen become blind, I am very hesitant to infer from this that any particular oxygen-exposed infant is afflicted. However, if I examine many oxygen-treated babies, I feel relatively sure that some of them are blind. My assurance increases with the number of observations about which I must form an opinion. In this class of events, there is uncertainty as to individuals, but as I include larger numbers in my assertions I attach greater weight to my inferences. It is with such classes of events (in which there are variations) and such inferences (in which there are uncertainties) that the science of probability is concerned.

It is useful to think of the kind of happening which we commonly encounter in medicine as a *series*. But it is a particular kind of series: one which combines individual irregularity and aggregate regularity. To return to my example, some infants exposed to oxygen become blind. If this statement is regarded simply as an indefinite proposition, the notion of a series does not seem obvious. It makes a statement about a certain unknown proportion of the whole, nothing more. However, the laws of probability are concerned not with indefinite propositions, but with numerical statements; they refer to a given proportion of the whole. And, with this latter conception it is difficult to avoid the idea of a series. What, for instance, is the meaning of the statement, One out of 20 infants exposed to oxygen becomes blind? It does not declare that in any given group of 20 oxygen-exposed infants, there will be one who becomes blind. The assertion incorporates the notion of results obtained in an examination of a long succession of oxygen-treated infants. And it implies that in this *series,* there will be a numerical proportion who are blind, not fixed and accurate at first, but which tends in the long run to approach 1 out of 20. This is the central idea of the probable-trend concept. It is necessary to envision a large number of observations or, as Venn emphasized, a *series* of them, if we are to use the power of the laws of probability to help with the interpretation of events in every-day experience. Inescapably, we come to a confrontation with the *seeming* capriciousness of the workings of chance. For, it turns out, the reasoning of the gambler (not as devil-may-care as he would have us believe) leads the way to a useful approach to the kinds of questions which bedevil physicians.

The simple coin-tossing game of "heads" and "tails" provides some clear illustrations of the fundamental principles of the theory of probability. The first thing to notice is that when a coin is thrown many times, the results of the successive tosses form a series. The separate throws (like the singly observed events in medicine) seem to occur chaotically, and the disorder gives rise to uncertainty. As long as we confine our attention to a few throws at a time, the series seems to be utterly irregular. But when we consider the overall results of a long succession, an order emerges. Finally, the pattern of chance is distinct and quite striking. In the game, there are runs of consecutive "heads" and of "tails," but the longer the play continues the less their relative proportion to the whole amounts involved; in the case of hundreds of throws of a coin the ratio of "heads" to "tails" will be very close to one-to-one. And, in a very large experience, runs of successive "heads" and "tails" also will approach fixed proportions. The point here is that in examining things and events in the natural world (those which occur in medicine and in coin-tossing) many of their qualities are variable. But their occurrence is quite predictable in the *aggregate* (see Gauss' Law in chapter notes). As a quality or attribute is noted in a long series, the proportion of occurrence is gradually subject to less variation and approaches some fixed value. Order gradually emerges out of disorder.

Obviously, there is an enormous difference between complex events in medicine and the straightforward occurrences in coin-tossing, but some similarities cannot be wished away. I must be quick to point out one difference which has practical significance. The gambler can calculate the probabilities of outcomes *before* making any real-world observations. He makes some reasonable assumptions:

1. There are an endless number of physical forces which may influence the outcome of each toss, but these are "indifferent," they do not align themselves in favor of either heads or tails (indeed, these are the motors of chance which operate haphazardly and account for the variation from toss to toss).
2. The outcome of each toss is an independent event (the coin has no "memory").
3. All of the possible and equally likely outcomes are obvious by inspecting the coin.

If these assumptions are correct, it is perfectly safe to declare that the probability for the outcome of "heads" (or "tails") at each toss is one-half. And a serious gambler can develop a betting strategy on the basis of calculations which predict the proportion of runs of successive "heads" (or "tails") which will be approached in an upcoming game. (The *a priori* computations—see chapter notes—indicate that in game-sets of 100 tosses, he can expect to find about 6 runs of two-heads-in-a-row, 3 runs of three-heads-in-a-row, and 1 run of four-heads-in-a-row; the expected frequencies of longer and rarer runs also can be calculated before the coin tossing commences.) When the results of a long series of *actual* tosses are inspected, the difference between the number of runs of heads expected by calculation and the number observed in fact provides the gambler with useful information. If the coin seems to defy the prediction consistently, this may lead to a betting scheme which takes advantage of the bias which is found.

The doctor is unable to calculate the "expected" proportions of occurrences of medical events in advance. Because of uncertainties about selection of observations and doubts about the independence of occurrences (for example, the concurrence of RLF in twins, see p 41), it is difficult to support the first two simplifying assumptions made by the gambler. And the third precondition is plainly impossible. In medicine, we cannot even imagine what an analysis of "all of the possible and equally likely outcomes" would mean, although we see very clearly what they mean in tossing a coin. In complex situations, we are obliged to substitute statistical probabilities, determined by experience. We note the variation in the occurrence of blindness and the "fixed proportion" which is approached in a long series of observations in infants who are treated with oxygen. *After* this information is in hand, we can make predictions with the same confidence as the coin-tossing gambler. The "regularities in the aggregate" make it possible to make inferences from "proportional propositions" (Venn's term). To return to my example again: Given that 1 infant in 20 treated with oxygen becomes blind, what can be inferred about the prospect in any particular infant? The reply can be couched in the same language used after calculating the *a priori* probabilities in coin-tossing: the odds for occurrence are close to those of obtaining runs of two-heads-in-a-row in a long series of tosses. Uncomfortable as it is (and far-fetched though it may seem to dwell on the analogy) here the resemblance between the gambler and the physician cannot be denied. Most importantly, the statistical probability of 1 in 20 found by experience may be compared with the proportion found in future series to search for the same kind of information which the gambler finds useful. The gambler's hopes for "doctored" coins which will defy the *a priori* calculations of outcome are exactly like the hopes of physicians for favorable treatments. Both dream of winning, but both are forced to test their fantasies in the real world of experience.

When the principles of the laws of chance were first taken up by agricultural scientists, the statistical techniques were not well suited to the needs of every-day research. Long series of observations were needed to estimate the frequency of occurrence of chance variations. For example, a plot of ground might be prepared with a new "treatment" and the subsequent yield from this plot found to be 10-percent higher than in an untreated field. The question would then arise as to how much confidence could be invested in the significance of a 10-percent difference in yields. Using the available statistical methods, it could be calculated, for instance, that 500 years' experience would be required to provide firm support for a distinction between the observed difference of 10 percent and the variations which occurred from year to year when the fields were treated uniformly. R. A. Fisher, who had been working for several years in the early 1920s with the laboratory staff at Rothamsted Experimental Station for Agricultural Research in Harpenden, England, became aware of the practical difficulties. What was required, he thought, was some sort of test of whether an apparent effect of treatment might be expected to occur reasonably often simply by chance; a test, furthermore, which did not require hopelessly large numbers of observations. He explored the mathematical implications of using small numbers of observations and he developed a practical plan for estimating the magnitude of variations in experiments that might be expected to occur by chance. Fisher proposed a design for field trials of treatments in which a plot of land was subdivided into blocks and within each block there was to be treated and untreated strips arranged in *random order*. The important point was that the results would now be governed entirely by the laws of chance. Each strip had an equal opportunity of treatment or no-treatment and each block was in fact a replicated trial. The replication now provided the estimate of chance variability (replacing the old direct-test-of-experience approach which frustrated researchers because of the need for a long series of annual yields). Additionally, the process of randomization secured the validity of the estimate of variations: "assignment-by-lot" ensured that the estimate was not biased ("loaded" would be the equivalent term in gambling). These principles of experimental design introduced by Fisher in the mid-1920s enabled experimenters to be free of the previous stringencies of large samples. The approach revolutionized the techniques of agricultural research throughout the world. Fisher's mathematical tests for small-sample problems (to estimate how often an observed result might be expected to occur by chance) were responsible for improvement in the efficiency of studies in many other fields of applied science, including medicine. Medical research workers began to use these new ideas, experimental designs, and mathematical tests in their own work, and some saw the relevance of the strategies to all medical studies.

For many years, however, the new movement was more evident in the laboratory than it was on the hospital ward.

The writings of A. Bradford Hill in England and Donald Mainland in Canada (and later in the United States) played a role in slowly overcoming the aversion of physicians to apply numerical methods in the interpretation of observations. Hill wrote a series of articles, prepared at the request of the editors of The Lancet in 1936, which described statistical methods that could be useful to physicians. The papers were published in book form a year later and the small volume quickly became a classic. A climate of awareness was gradually created which paved the way for the 1946 debut of a distinctive form of bedside research: the randomized clinical trial.

The episode was triggered by the discovery that a new drug, streptomycin, was effective in the treatment of experimental tuberculosis in guinea pigs. Shortly after, in 1945 and 1946, the drug was used in human tuberculosis in the United States; the results were encouraging, but inconclusive. Only a small supply of streptomycin was available in England and the British Medical Research Council was faced with the problem of how to proceed with the scant amount allocated to it for research purposes. (Most of the country's supply was taken up for two rapidly fatal forms of disease: miliary and meningeal tuberculosis.) The Council decided that its cache would best be employed in a rigorously planned investigation with concurrent controls. (I find it quite interesting that limited resources played a role in initiating this model of caution and safety from the patient's point of view, and of moral responsibility and scientific excellence from the community's perspective.) After considerable planning beginning in September 1946, a committee (including A. Bradford Hill) decided to limit the trial to tuberculous patients with closely defined features: acute progressive infection, diagnosis proven by bacteriologic test, status unsuitable for collapse treatment (injection of air into the pleural cavity to collapse and, thus, "rest" the lung), and age 15–25 years. Up to the time of the proposed trial, bed rest was considered to be the only suitable form of treatment for a patient with these charcteristics. After a detailed protocol of procedures was drawn up, patients were recruited from the London area and beyond. The first patients to be accepted (by a panel of physicians) were admitted to designated centers in January 1947. By September of that year, 109 persons were enrolled: 2 patients died within a preliminary week of observation, leaving 107 in the trial. At the end of a week of observation for each patient, assignment to treatment was made by opening a sealed envelope drawn from a set provided for each center (the sequence of assignments in the envelopes had been prearranged in an unpredictable order determined from tables of random numbers); 55 were allotted to the streptomycin group and 52 to the bed-rest group. Patients in both groups remained in bed for at least 6 months and the outcomes were assessed at the end of that period. Fifty-one of the 55 patients treated with streptomycin and 38 of 52 who were treated with bed rest were alive at the end of 6 months. The difference in outcome between the two groups was declared "statistically significant": a variation in survival of this size would be expected to occur purely-by-chance less often than one time in a hundred.

It is worth examining the unstated assumptions which underlie the langauge used in the concluding statement of this pioneering study. The declaration envisioned that in a very large series of tuberculous patients who received the standard treatment, bed rest, the proportion of survivors at the end of a 6-month observation period would be subject to a certain variability as the result of a number of unknown factors (the play of chance). In order to estimate the size of these variations, the committee modelled the design of the trial on Fisher's strategy of random assignment to treatments. The variability in outcome *expected* in bed-rest-treated patients was compared with the *observed* outcome in streptomycin-treated patients, and the question which was posed had the same form as Fisher's questions in the 1920s: What reason is there to think that the relatively small group of 55 patients who received streptomycin might not have experienced a higher rate of survival even without this treatment? The committee applied the mathematical techniques of analysis which had been worked out for small-sample problems in agricultural research to determine if the observed difference in the trial was more than would be likely to arise merely as a fluke. And the declaration of "statistical significance" was couched in the grammer of chance. The terms were familiar to any gambler: streptomycin treatment was a fairly good bet. (In *repeated* randomized trials involving 107 patients, one could expect to win 99 percent of the time; this is the equivalent of betting against four heads in a row in *repeated* games of coin tossing.) It is important to consider the limits of the conclusions which were made at the end of the streptomycin trial. Notice that the committee made no claim that the efficacy of streptomycin treatment had been *proven* by the experience of treating 55 patients. Also, there was very little assurance that the observed survival rate (93 percent) would hold up in future experience. In fact, there was every reason to expect that the survival rate with streptomycin treatment would be subject to the influence of least as many unknown factors as in bed-rest treatment. A large number of observations of outcomes among future groups of patients treated with the new drug was needed to estimate the "fixed proportion"; an indication of the efficiency of the new treatment.

The conservative tone of the statements which were made by the Research Council's committee stands in quiet contrast to the extravagant claims made in some of the reports which I reviewed in Chapter 10. And it is also worth noting that the doctors who carried out the carefully planned study were conscious of their responsibility to obtain as much information as possible from the rare experience of a formal comparison, which might never be repeated in the management of pulmonary tuberculosis. In addition to the enumeration of survivors, systematic comparisons were made of every facet of the course of the illness in the two groups. The study provided a wealth of descriptive information, not only about the beneficial effects of streptomycin, but also its limitations (for instance, drug treatment did not close large cavities in the lung) and toxicity (detrimental effects on the vestibular apparatus of the ear). The planning committee noted at the end of the trial that the need for a control group was underscored by the finding of impressive improvement in some patients treated by bed rest alone. The streptomycin trial was the first controlled clinical investigation of its kind (which led to a positive result—see chapter notes). It was followed by a long series of pathfinding clinical trials conducted by the Medical Research Council which evaluated a wide variety of proposed treatments.

The format of present-day trials using the technique of randomized controls evolved from the British experiences. Until recently, the mathematical strategies for statistical analysis tended to receive more attention than was given to the basic logical concepts of the design of trials. In the past few years, however, Feinstein has examined, in minute detail, the conceptual "architecture" of studies involving free-willed physicians and their free-living patients. From his analyses, and those of Sackett, the methodologic discipline has advanced considerably (Appendix D). In planning bedside studies, unlike laboratory experiments, a host of real-world (potentially biasing) influences must be taken into account.

Valid comparison is the *sine qua non* of a trial of a new treatment. If past events are to be used as a standard of comparison, it must be presumed that everything except the new treatment has remained uniform with the passage of time. Under such circumstances it is unnecessary to use the ponderous machinery of the experimental method since the observational approach provides interpretable information. This was exemplified by the experience with tuberculous infection of the meningeal membranes enveloping the brain: prior to 1946, it had been uniformly fatal. Biologic and environmental factors had no known effect on the outcome of this form of tuberculosis. The results of prior treatments did not vary; patients of all ages, either sex, with or without other complications, etc. all succumbed.

When streptomycin was first used to treat a series of patients with this disorder, it was unnecessary to go beyond the step of Claude Bernard's "active observations" (". . . made with a preconceived idea, with intention to verify the accuracy of a mental conception."). And, the results of the consecutive-treatments approach were secure (since the premise, "all untreated patients die," was true). A single instance of survival was clear evidence of the effectiveness of treatment. However, a large series was required for an estimate of the variability in survival rate (now the efficiency of treatment was influenced by innumerable biologic and environmental factors). And, in studies to determine whether a new treatment was superior to streptomycin, all of the problems with variability would emerge. As I have emphasized repeatedly, inevitable effects in medicine are rare. Most bedside experiences are of the kind I have described in this book. They are far from invariant, and they are beset with interpretive difficulties. It was this background of experience which accounted for the general uncertainty about the reports from Melbourne and Birmingham (Figs. 4-1 and 4-2) concerning the role of supplemental oxygen in RLF. The skepticism which greeted the first suggestions was a responsible reaction on the part of the medical community as a whole and of individual physicians who were concerned about the well-being of their patients. What could be made of the finding that the frequency of RLF in a nursery fell from 3 out of 13 in 1944– 50 (with "high oxygen") to 0 out of 6 in 1951 (with "low oxygen"). Here, the guidance concerning a hierarchy of evidence provided by Claude Bernard was helpful. For, it is clear that the association found by this "active" observation was a higher order of evidence than the association noted in the previous "passive" observation (the Boston observations concerning RLF, iron, and vitamins had been made by sifting through past records; the observers were not led to the observation by a preconceived idea). Moreover, the pitifully small numbers did not detract from the *qualitative* strength of the English evidence. The point is that this was in essence a *single* "active" observation: it advanced the state of knowledge by one notch. The report of the Texas air-lock experience (p 72) quoted very large denominators (the death rate fell from 1.9 percent among 6324 births in 1949 to 1.5 percent among 1372 births in 1950 in association with use of the device), but it also advanced the state of knowledge by one notch. The Houston experience was, in essence, a single active observation. Now, I do not wish to denigrate the *potential* importance of the Birmingham report, the air-lock report, and all of the accounts of "active observations" which I have cited in this volume (including, I must emphasize, the announcement that 28 infants improved dramatically following epsom-salt enemas, p 87). For, in each instance the observed associations were made with a preconceived idea, and they provided leads to the solutions of very important problems. Moreover, each lead made it possible to frame a question in the form of a "proportional proposition." Instead of, "Can low oxygen treatment reduce the risk of RLF?," after the Birmingham observation the question was quantified: "Can low oxygen reduce the risk of RLF from about 20 percent to almost zero?" After the Houston report, the question was "Can use of the air-lock reduce mortality from ca. 2 percent to ca. 1.5 percent", and so it was in all of the reports of "active observations." What needs to be understood is that the numbers provided in each of these reports served the important function of converting the indefinite propositions into a form which could be dealt with by the resolving power of the laws of probability. But the numerical differences provided no quantitative information about how often such differences could be expected purely by chance. The "how often" information could only be obtained safely and reliably by an additional step-up in the hierarchal process which seeks to protect patients and improve understanding. A formal test was required of the question *How often* would the apparent association between low oxygen and a fall in RLF frequency from ca 20 percent to almost zero be expected simply by chance? The direct-test-of-experience would entail a long series of observations in groups of identically treated infants (preferably in different hospitals) to obtain an estimate of expected variations; this was the backdrop against which a 20 percent-to-zero change would have to be viewed. (The need for evidence from different institutions was quite important. The populations of patients in any one hospital was so highly selected there could be little confidence that a specific experience would give a reliable estimate. Recall that results observed after lowering oxygen in Birmingham and Oxford in England, Melbourne, and Paris were widely discrepant.) I cannot emphasize this point enough: the magnitude of the interpretive difficulties in the direct-experience test is much greater in bedside medicine than is found in most other fields of inquiry. Hopelessly large numbers of observations are required because the "background" fluctuations are usually large and the outcome differences are relatively small (in medicine we are usually trying to decide about a small change, i.e., from 73 to 93 percent survival, as in the pulmonary tuberculosis trial in England, rather than the striking change in the tuberculous meningitis experience, i.e., from no survivors without streptomycin to 81-percent survival with treatment).

The important contribution of R. A. Fisher to the development of scientific methodology was the novel *design* of experiments; he did not perform feats of mathematical legerdemain. The statistical techniques which he invented (and earlier mathematical tools which originated with Karl Pearson) were not meant·to be used like recipes out of a cookbook in the hope of extracting meaning from any and all sets of numbers derived from unplanned observations. Tests of statistical significance, Mainland stressed, are not magical maneuvers for determining whether there is some hidden bias in an experiment. The conduct of an investigation must be so *designed* as to minimize the likelihood of systematic "loading" of extraneous factors which will influence the outcomes. If the precautions have not been taken *in advance,* the mathematical tests are simply inapplicable. For instance, it is misleading to perform statistical arithmetic on the numbers obtained in the Melbourne observations (Table 13-1). A declaration of "statistical significance" is meaningless because infants in each of the three hospitals did not have an equal opportunity of treatment with "high" or with "moderate" oxygen. (The key requirement of Fisherian design was not fulfilled: random assignment of treatments to ensure that the results would now be governed entirely by the laws of chance.) The same problem arose in interpreting the initial results in RLF outcome after ACTH treatments (Table 13-1). Again, only assignments-by-lot *within* each hospital could satisfy the equal opportunity assumption needed for use of the statistical tests (and, as this experience demonstrated, this is a basic requirement for the protection of patients). The 1953–54 Cooperative Study of RLF subsequently confirmed the "lead" which was indicated by the relatively small difference in RLF frequency observed in Melbourne hospitals. On the other hand, our randomized controlled trial of ACTH failed to confirm the striking difference in results found in the two New York hospitals. Before

Table 13-1

Two "Leads" Concerning RLF (1950–1951)

"Active Observations"			RLF Occurrence	Difference
Melbourne				
One "high-oxygen" hospital (123 infants)	vs	Two "moderate-oxygen" hospitals (58 infants)	19% vs 7%	− 12%*
New York				
No treatment Lincoln Hospital (7 infants)	vs	ACTH Babies Hospital (31 infants)	86% vs 19%	− 67%**

*Supported by subsequent controlled trial.
**Refuted by subsequent controlled trial.

the controlled trials were conducted there was simply no way to know which of the initial favorable leads in the two countries was false.

I do not wish to minimize the practical difficulties of conducting clinical studies with *concurrent* controls. But hardship alone cannot account for the fact that the basic requisites of design are met in a very small proportion of present-day studies which assess the efficacy (and the risks!) of new treatments. There is a persistent "straw-man" issue: the multiplicity of clinical variables. Many physicians believe that comparisons of treatments using concurrent controls are impractical in clinical medicine because it is almost impossible to assemble two groups that are matched exactly in every clinical detail. I find it hard to understand how this belief supports the validity of using past events as a standard of comparison. But this aside, the argument reveals a fundamental lack of understanding about the role of randomization. Fisher explained that it is pointless to insist that all the conditions in compared groups must be exactly alike. This is an impossible requirement in all biologic experimentation because the list of possible factors which might influence the outcome can never be exhausted: *the number is unknown.* It is random assignment of treatments which serves as the fundamental safeguard under these conditions of uncertainty about risk variables (an inescapable condition of medical studies). And, to repeat, scattering-by-chance guarantees the validity of the test of significance by which the results of the trial are judged.

I would be unfair if I suggested that the resistance to lottery-like proceedings is due entirely to lack of awareness of the logical basis for the precautions. Once more, there are some emotional issues to consider. The thought of random allocation to treatments in which blindness or life are at stake, is, at first flush, a repugnant one. I believe the revulsion is an all-too-human denial of reality: chance is in control of our lives to an extent which is too uncomfortable to dwell upon. Bronowski pointed out that the early readers of *The Origin of Species* were outraged, in their religious and their moral convictions, by the central place of chance in Darwin's theory of evolution. I suspect it is religion-based morality which stands behind the self-righteous statements I have heard in courtrooms. But, I hasten to add, the unease is deep-seated. Despite all evidence indicating the enormous risks of guessing in medicine, we are all prone to feel that a well-meaning guess is somehow not as cold and unfeeling as the flip of a coin. I can recall very vividly, when we were conducting the formal evaluation of ACTH treatment, that one of my colleagues refused to allow his patient to be enrolled in the trial. He was convinced that the treatment was effective and he proceeded to administer ACTH to his patient who had very early signs of RLF. I can also recall, sadly, the fatal infection which occurred as a complication of that treatment. Another example of the unwillingness of physicians to consider that their attentions may be dangerous was related by Cochrane. It occurred in England during an attempt to evaluate intensive-care units for patients with coronary artery heart disease. He found a considerable vested interest in the results of a randomized controlled trial to compare the outcome in coronary-care units versus care at home. The first report of the trial showed a slightly higher death rate in hospitalized patients than among patients treated at home. Someone reversed the figures and showed them to a coronary-care-unit enthusiast. He immediately declared that the trial was unethical and must be stopped at once. However, when he was shown the correct results, he could not be persuaded to declare the hospital units unethical!

I find it completely understandable that compassionate physicians, struggling for solutions to unsolved medical problems, form emotional attachments to leads which develop during the search. And I do not scoff at these feelings; but I do argue that they should not be hidden. When personal predilections are openly expressed, it is easier to design a test plan which will keep these from entering into treatment decisions. The issue of "experimenter's bias" was brought home to me in an early (fruitless) trial of the effect of artificial light on the occurrence of RLF. Assignment to "light" or "no-light" was made on the basis of blue and white marbles in a box. One day, I noticed that our head nurse reached into the box for a marble and then replaced it because it wasn't the color that corresponded to her belief about the best treatment for her babies. I became convinced that we had to shift to sealed envelopes, as used in the British streptomycin trial. When the first sealed envelope was drawn, the resident physician held it up to the light to see the assignment inside! I took the envelopes home and my wife and I wrapped each assignment-sticker in black paper and resealed the envelopes.

What is the alternative to assignments-by-lot in formal testing? Unfortunately, formats which depend on physician-prescribed assignments are not satisfactory. For, if doctors were sufficiently prescient to choose correctly among unknowns, the sad record of the past would not be there to haunt us. Nonetheless, the resistance to randomization as a method of allocating patients to treatment has given rise to proposals for "adaptive" designs (using information obtained during the course of the trial to determine the treatment assignment for the next patient). Some of these adaptive procedures have been given colorful names (e.g., "play the winner", "two-arm bandit strategy") and they have attracted considerable interest.

But the outcomes of treatments are often not evident until some time has passed; in the history of perinatal treatments, short-term "winners" have sometimes become long-term "losers." This point is illustrated by the Cooperative Study of RLF; it was one of the first attempts to use an adaptive approach. Only one-third of the infants were assigned to routine unrestricted oxygen in the intial three months of the study to evaluate survival differences under the oxygen regimens. The favorable short-term results (no *apparent* difference in mortality) of this first phase of the study (involving 212 infants) indicated that it was safe to proceed with curtailed oxygen for the remaining nine months (an additional 574 infants were enrolled). The long-term results of curtailment of oxygen in this very large number of infants were never evaluated. But, as I have indicated (p 64) there is reason to suspect that there were unfavorable late effects. A review of recent methodologic alternatives to randomized trials concluded that the latter type of clinical investigation is very complex, expensive, and time-consuming; but the format remains as the most useful tool which has been devised for comparisons of treatments.

I wish to comment on the myth that patients enrolled in a randomized trial are called upon to take unwarranted risks for the sake of others. The issue becomes inflamed when babies are involved. Despite all evidence from past experience which demonstrates that unsuspected risks of innovation can be minimized by the controlled-trial strategy, the distorted notion persists. Chalmers objected to the assumption that there was greater interest in future patients than in enrollees. An equal case can be made, he noted, for randomization to result in a *better* chance that a patient will receive the proper treatment. Our experience with sulfisoxazole (p 80) was a convincing illustration of his view. Additionally, a task force of the Department of Health, Education and Welfare undertook a systematic attempt in 1976 to estimate the nature and magnitude of the risk for human subjects who participate in research projects. A survey of 538 medical researchers, involving about 39,000 patients, indicated that the risks in therapeutic trials were no greater than those of treatment in other settings.

Another aspect of this "unjustified-risk" argument arises when it is suggested that controlled trials of promising treatments are unwarranted in conditions of very high mortality; severe hyaline-membrane disease has been used as an example. This is completely logical if the arguments are confined to the category of inevitably fatal conditions (as I noted above, in tuberculous meningitis). But the situation is rarely this simple. A Boston group observed that patients with severe and fatal disease merely represent the "tip of an iceberg." There are almost always many more with milder forms of the same disease, and increased interest in diagnosis takes place when a new treatment is introduced. This invariably leads to the recognition of less severe examples which were previously overlooked. Consequently, outcome in currently treated patients appears improved, even when the treatment is without effect or actually deleterious. The incident involving epsom-salt enemas to treat hyaline-membrane disease was a tragic example of this phenomenon.

Legal issues surrounding the matter of random assignment of treatments were reviewed by Fried in 1974. He concluded that the law is incomplete on most of the difficult dilemmas posed (e.g., informing patients of the fact of randomization and whether or not randomization does violence to the duty a doctor owes his patient). He also discussed the matter of values (". . . the question of what is right in principle") in considerable detail and he made a plea for increased candor, education and participation in the planning and conduct of randomized clinical trials. I believe there is an enormous gulf which separates the law and medicine in these matters. One indication of the semantic distance between the disciplines is seen in use of the word "experimentation"; in the courts the term connotes malpractice (procedures which vary from accepted practice).

A series of important questions about the issue of properly designed studies to evaluate proposed treatments was posed by Kabat:

Is it ethical to do a study on human subjects with a design such that one may come up with the wrong answer? Is it fair to the participants? Is it fair to those who subsequently become the recipients or victims of what becomes a prescribed but useless prophylactic or therapeutic measure? Once a large-scale field trial has yielded a conclusion, right or wrong, and becomes official and sacrosanct, how many potentially better studies will not be carried out because of it? How much of a false sense of security will it give patients, their families and society? Suppose the conclusion was reached because of inadequate controlled experimentation?"

Viewed with the hindsight of almost a quarter of a century, I see the Cooperative Study of RLF as an example of the very situation envisioned by Kabat. The trial did not provide a wrong answer, but it came up with an incomplete answer. And once the results were announced, it became unthinkable to test the unexpected leads which were found. (Recall that the Cooperative Study had not been designed to test the relationships between *varying* durations of oxygen exposure, *varying* concentrations of supplemental oxygen and RLF. The associations described in the final report had been disclosed by "data-dredging": the mass of information collected in the study was inspected in a search for correlates. The finding that duration rather than concentration of oxygen correlated with RLF-risk constituted an untested hypothesis. And the provisional quality of this *ex post facto* evidence was the same as that found in so many of the previous analytic surveys: associations which had failed to pass a critical test.) However, when it became possible to measure the state of oxygenation of blood in the 1960s, the unresolved issues were approachable. Now a question of trade-off of risks could be posed: Can the risk of brain damage and death be reduced substantially, at the cost of a minimum increase in the risk of RLF, if oxygen is administered in amounts to maintain oxygen in the blood at the upper part of the so-called "normal" range rather than low "normal" (see p 60)? I mentioned earlier that a Cooperative Study was undertaken in 1969 to explore the relationship between blood oxygen and RLF risk; however, the design of the study doomed it from the start. Measurements were made of oxygen in the blood of infants who received supportive treatment according to individual-physician prescription (the "active" observations approach) rather than by random assignment to prescribed conditions of blood oxygen (the experimental approach). At the end of 8 years of effort (3 years of observations and 5 years of analysis of the results!), there were no interpretable findings. To this day, when oxygen is administered to premature infants, they are exposed to the intertwined risks of brain damage, death and RLF with nothing more than authoritative guessing as protection.

It is painful to hear some of the questions raised in malpractice suits against conscientious physicians who treated infants prior to September 1954. One question in particular reveals the gulf of misunderstanding between medicine and community; it is, On what *day* was the truth concerning the association between oxygen treatment and the risk of RLF established? The accusatory climate created by this kind of absolutist thinking has had the ruinous effect of downgrading the role of doubt in medicine. ·And, the combined resistance of social, political and ethical forces to the use of the experimental method in studies involving children has encouraged a return to the hazards of Galenist reasoning. Somehow, the community must come to the realization that excellence in medical research is to be fostered as a public safety measure. Even a society made wary of science, because of the misapplication of technical developments, must know that the underlying logical machinery of the scientific method is in the public interest. Science, Popper noted, is one of the very few human activities in which errors are systematically criticized, and fairly often, in time, corrected.

14

The Future for Studies Involving American Children

Doubtless ye will say unto me this parable, Physician, heal thyself.

Luke iv, 23

I have no prescription to cure the enigmatic social dysfunctions which have been outlined, and I have no intention of proposing palliatives to ease the pain. The problem-set of complex societal issues concerning research involving children in the United States does not lend itself to an inspirational solution. I do not agree with those who are seeking make-shift compromises to calm the fears of critics and allow everything to return to "normal." Price has suggested that the present crisis of attitudes toward all research is an inevitable consequence of the characteristics of the growth curve of science as a whole, which has had a long life of purely exponential growth (Fig. 14-1). As this pattern of increase reaches the midpoint of the "natural" curve and enters a period of secession from the accustomed conditions of expansion, there is increasing concern over the problems of manpower, publication, and expenditure that demand solution by reorganization. If Price is correct, these are inescapable phenomena associated with the approach of the upper limit of scientific escalations. "If we expect to discourse in scientific style about science, and to plan accordingly," he

145

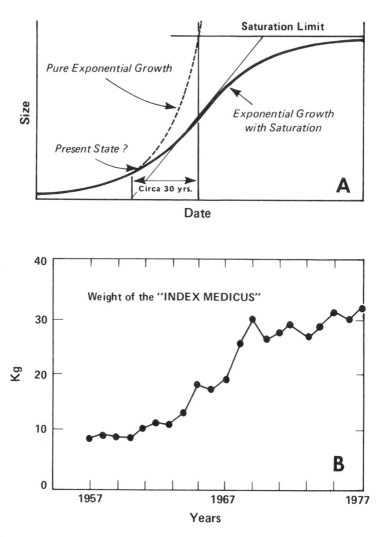

Fig. 14-1. A. General form of the logistic growth curve of science in the United States described by Price. The steady state of exponential growth is followed by a decline to linear growth and finally an exponential rate of deceleration. He estimated that only about 30 years must elapse (from the "present state" in 1959) between the period when some few percent of difficulty is felt and the time when that trouble has become so acute that it cannot possibly be satisfied. B. The "growth curve" of medical knowledge estimated by Durack from the weight of the annual volumes of *Index Medicus* (the National Library of Medicine's bibliography of the literature of biomedicine).

146

writes, "we shall have to call this approaching period [of the involvement of science with society] . . . Stable Saturation; if we have no such hopes, we must call it senility."

There is a special need to seek stability in the relationships between perinatal research activities and the community-at-large. Anything which influences the quantity and quality of human reproduction has a magnified social impact (the term "environmental impact," used in other contexts, is not entirely inappropriate here); as I said earlier, the effects extend well beyond the current generation. Health care development in perinatal medicine is, in essence, a political and social process; more than in any other field of medicine, there must be public participation in defining the goals of the medical effort. And there should be community evaluation of progress. An advisory panel to the Department of Health, Education and Welfare reviewed the question of whether or not policies (in the 1970s) to protect the rights of patients participating in government-supported health research were satisfactory. They concluded that it is the spirit in which our society undertakes the use of human beings for research which will determine the protection they receive. And the panelists urged much greater participation by society in the decisions which influence so many lives. Eisenberg has advised that there will be moral gain as well as health gain if we can create a community of shared responsibility for health research. An example of the kind of cooperative effort which is possible when there is unusually high motivation occurred in the polio vaccine trials conducted in the United States in 1954. Poliomyelitis had been one of the most dreaded diseases of childhood. But the fears were out of proportion to its total impact in children as compared, say, with automobile accidents. Nonetheless, it appeared in recurrent, seasonal waves, leaving many crippled children in their wake, and the threat of major epidemic outbreaks of the disorder was very frightening. American determination to combat this infectious condition was bolstered by the fact that President Franklin D. Roosevelt had been paralyzed as the result of polio acquired in early adult life. His former law partner, Basil O'Connor, led national campaigns to raise money for research to prevent or cure the disease. These fund-raising efforts supported investigations leading to Ender's method of cultivating the polio virus in the chick embryo and to the development of the Salk vaccine. The hoped-for preventive measure was ready in 1954 to be field tested in trials involving school children. The object of the trials was to evaluate effectiveness of immunization in preventing the disorder and to detect any unforeseen complications of the vaccine. News reports explained these objectives and described the research methodology *before* the trials were begun. Health departments electing use of the experimental approach enrolled 401, 974 children; parental permission for participation was obtained and children received either Salk vaccine or ineffective salt solution as decided by random ordering (each assignment remained undisclosed until outcomes in all children were reported). Among 200,745 children in the vaccinated group, the rate of polio was 0.028 percent (of these 58 percent had paralytic complications, and there were no deaths); among 201,229 in the control group, polio developed in 0.071 percent (of these, paralytic complications occurred in 81 percent, and death occurred in 1.4 percent of those affected).

The polio vaccine trials demonstrated that when the American public perceives that it is threatened by a frightening "enemy," there is whole hearted support and *active* participation, including the involvement of children as subjects in research trials. Although the vaccine-trials episode was a landmark in the history of communion between medical researchers and the public, paradoxically, the spectacular success of the effort has had some unfortunate after-effects. The polio experience raised expectations about medical omnipotence which were unreal, and it has led to enormous pressure for quick solutions to long-standing problems, notably in perinatal medicine. (The National Foundation–March of Dimes, organized for the efforts against polio, is now directing its attention to congenital malformations and other perinatal problems.) Regrettably, the uniqueness of the issues in problems of pregnancy and the newborn period have been inadequately stressed. Simply stated, the scientific evidence needed for decision-making must be of a higher order of completeness and credibility than that generated in the vaccine trials. Poliomyelitis, as I said, was a relatively uncommon disorder of childhood in the 1950s; it was responsible for 6 percent of all deaths in children; it crippled far fewer individuals, and the social consequences were not as far-reaching as the conditions which complicate pregnancy and delivery; importantly, there were no questions in polio survivors about the transmission of heritable defects to future generations, and there was no reason to suspect that the long-term cost to human society might wipe out the short-term gains. The stakes involved in decisions about interventions in perinatal matters are considerably higher than those which had to be considered in recommending a national policy for polio vaccination. Even in retrospect, the contrast between the extent of the successes achieved by the 1953–54 oxygen trial for RLF and the 1954 vaccine trials for polio does not convey fully the difference in magnitude and complexity of the two problems. Let me be understood. If the search for comprehension in matters concerning human procreation is to be more democratic, more thorough, and safer than in the past, it follows that innovations should be applied more slowly, and on a more limited scale than heretofore. These words may appear to be cheerless to those with a millenarian outlook who wish to see the solution to all of the outstanding problems in their lifetime. They may seem heartless to parents who wish to see a solution to a specific problem within their child's lifetime. But I hope my formulation does not sound strange to those who value a search for the truth. For, I am not advising a reduction in the volume of basic biomedical research, and I strongly reject the notion that all laboratory research must be directed toward a specific clinical goal. (A review was made recently of the key observations which led to the ten most important advances in cardiovascular and pulmonary medicine and surgery in the last 30 years. Research efforts which had no foreseeable bearing on these clinical problems—the non-goal-directed investigations—paid off in terms of key discoveries almost twice as handsomely as other types of research and development combined.) I argue that the pace should slow at the *threshold of bedside applications* of proposals which arise from the findings in biomedical studies. My advice is exactly the opposite to the activist viewpoint which has been called the "Lyndon Johnson doctrine," after his 1966 speech chiding the research community for its alleged failure to translate the findings of basic research speedily into practice. Proposed interventions, I contend, should be evaluated in cautious, graded steps, adhering to the same standard of scientific rigor used in preclinical research. But these *applications* should be sharply goal-directed. Overall progress in medicine is not measured by the rate of change, but the rate of advancement toward a goal. And, to repeat, the goal in perinatal interventions must *not* be defined exclusively by physicians. The limits of medical action have been clearly demarcated by Freidson: the conduct of medical practice or application of expertise is analytically distinct from expertise or knowledge itself. The distinction makes it clear that when decisions are fundamentally moral or evaluative rather than substantive, laymen have as much if not more to contribute to them than have experts. This assumption reflects the substance of equality in a free society, Freidson emphasized, equality not of ability, knowledge or means, but moral equality. Medicine must restore this balance if it is to reverse a disturbing trend: it is becoming an institution of social control.

The era of society's involvement with science can begin when there is public realization that science values a search for understanding about the natural world. The search will become a source of American social values only when our society accepts the assumption that no belief will survive if it conflicts with factual evidence. The medical research community takes it for granted that it should pursue the truth, that the truth is still being pursued, and that the pursuit will go on always. The truth has not already been found. Bronowski pointed out that a society that believes that the truth is at hand, for example in politics or religion, simply imposes it; it is an authoritarian society. I believe as medicine moves away from its authoritarian past and becomes more scientific, it should abandon the "breakthrough" mentality (a "Eureka! We have found it!" warp which began with the discoveries of penicillin and polio vaccine). Physicians should become concerned with the continuing *process* of the search for understanding. There should be a heightened emphasis on the adequacy of the design of research. Medawar detected such movement in a review of the development of the scientific method over the past 300 years: inductive experiments to increase the store of factual information (of the type advised by Francis Bacon—through careful observation of a number of individual cases, a scientist hoped to "induce" a general statement about all cases) are being replaced by critical experiments carried out to test hypotheses or preconceived ideas. In the latter type of experiment, which seeks to discriminate among possibilities, problems of design are placed before those of validation. A similar trend in the use of the scientific method in clinical investigations is more difficult to perceive. For example, a recent review of the acceptance of the randomized clinical trial as the method of choice for evaluating clinical treatments indicated very slow progress. The experimental format rose from 0.3 percent of studies testing treatments in gastroenterology in 1964 to 1.7 percent in 1973. The authors concluded that randomized clinical trials would take over completely by the year 2010 provided the increase is exponential; in about 700 years if it is linear. An interview survey of 61 institutions conducting research in children (July 1974–June 1975) reported that random assignment methodology was used in about 1 out of 6 clinical studies (among 219 projects in which the investigators answered the question posed).

What can be done about improperly designed studies involving human subjects—studies that cannot possibly yield interpretable results? I have argued throughout this book that improvement in scientific rigor inevitably results in improved protection for the participants in medical studies. And a remedy suggests itself from the historical trend in the development of the scientific method: an increased preoccupation with methodology. Editors and review committees of medical journals have it within their power to prescribe a cure: a change in the primary criterion for acceptance of reports describing bedside studies, from an emphasis on *results* to an insistence on proper *design*. Walster and Cleary found a similar problem with studies in the social sciences and they proposed a new editorial policy for articles which make inferential statistical analyses of results. The cardinal rule in experimental design, they argued, is that any decision regarding the treatment of data must be made *prior* to the inspection of the data. If this rule is extended to publication decisions, it follows that when an article is submitted for review, the data and the results should be withheld. This would guarantee that the decision to publish, or not to publish, would be unrelated to the outcome of the research. The editorial decision would be based upon such factors as the adequacy of the design, and the relevance of the research to theoretical and topical issues. Radical as this proposal sounds at first hearing, it is quite logical and entirely practical. I believe the plan deserves serious consideration.

The challenge for the future in clinical studies involving babies is to develop acceptable processes for changing the ordered pattern of response to new proposals: formal evaluation should be undertaken before, not after, wide use of new treatments and procedures. However, there should be improvements in the approach which relate to scientific and to democratic principles (and the two are not antithetical, they are complementary). I believe small-scale explorations of various approaches (experiments in the procedure of bedside experimentation) are in order, and I wish to make several proposals which might be considered in a search for improvements. These are related to public involvement and concerns in clinical studies, the categorization of risks and benefits, a schema for informed surveillance in clinical trials, and, finally, a Popperian approach to experimental tactics.

Clinical studies have been conducted more frequently among impoverished minorities than among the privileged American classes. The poor became subjects on whom studies were done because of their convenience (researchers were located in the teaching hospitals used by poor patients) and because of gross insensitivity to the unfairness of the practice. To the extent that the disadvantaged young were not representative of all American children, the sampling bias in the past was an example of poor science *and* poor democracy. The National Commmission for the Protection of Human Subjects of Biomedical and Behavioral Research (established by an act of Congress in 1974) has recently advised that children who participate in research projects should be selected so that the burdens of participation are distributed equitably among the segments of our society. But how is this to be accomplished? Volunteering thwarts the basic principle of random sampling (the latter is used to *assure* equality of representation), and there are gross social inequitites. For example, Jonas advised that the general criteria for participants in clinical experimentation should include the very qualities least likely to be found among those on the lowest rungs of the social ladder: a maximum of identification, understanding and spontaneity. Researchers should look for subjects among the most highly motivated, the most highly educated, and the least "captive" members of the community, he advised. These qualities describe physicians and their families, but it has been my long and consistent experience that they are unwilling to allow their own children and grandchildren to participate in research projects. It seems to me that conscription-by-lot, however unpopular, is an honorable solution to the dilemma posed by the Commission's recommendation. Jonas discussed this approach and rejected it on the grounds that it was an unacceptable philosophy. Indeed, he viewed it as threatening and utopian, an approach from which we should recoil. I appreciate his horror, but I suggest that it stems from the popular (pejorative) opinion that the subjects in human investigations must undertake unwarranted risks. If, on the other hand, systematic bedside research is viewed realistically, as the only practical means for protecting individuals from unknown risks in medicine, perhaps the rejection may not be quite so final. Democratic societies have used a draft to choose young men to defend the populace against real and imagined enemies, and medical warfare is no less real. Obviously, extensive educational efforts will be required to convince Americans that unassessed changes in care-taking practices may produce effects that are as devastating as the consequences of enemy action in war. But a glance at the numbers of infants who died or who were left blind, brain damaged or malformed in modern treatment disasters should be sobering: the totals are greater than in the polio epidemics—they rival wartime statistics!

Similar heroic and more specific efforts will be required to convince Americans that the under-utilized randomized clinical trial is the most powerful defensive weapon against the backfire of modern arms in medical arsenals. Although I argue that the educational efforts should be undertaken, I know that it will not be easy. Scientifically rigorous clinical study is slow and doctors in the front-lines of medical practice are under enormous pressure to "do something." For example, the early observations that supplemental oxygen appeared to be useful in the management of premature infants made it very difficult for experienced physicians and nurses to consider testing effects which they found to be self-evident. Conscientious doctors, confronted with the problems of pneumonia in newborn infants (complicating the influenza epidemics in the 1950s), felt they could not wait for the results of a formal trial of the effectiveness and safety of chloramphenicol. But if these undisciplined approaches are to change, public pressure on physicians must change. A call for action should take into account that the modern doctor is more like a weapons specialist manning the push-button console of a missile launcher than a romantic warrior armed with a sword. Modern conditions call for cautious tactics: limited forays and planned battles against ignorance concerning medical matters. Simple concern for the public interest dictates that we can no longer ignore Claude Bernard's maxim: science teaches us to doubt and, in ignorance, to refrain.

The classification of clinical investigations into two arbitrary categories ("therapeutic" and "nontherapeutic", see p 117) is an illusory dichotomy which encourages subterfuge. Guidelines for the conduct of studies prepared by the American Academy of Pediatrics in 1977 attempt to distinguish between the indistinct classes; but the set of recommendations proposed by the National Commission abandons the distinction. I believe that in all studies, regardless of the purported intent, the relationships between risks and benefits should be considered on a continuous scale. At one end of the range there are procedures with virtually no benefit which should be balanced by practically no risk; at the other extreme the risks are so great that they outweigh any conceivable benefit. In addition, I suggest that categories of risks and benefits should be weighted differentially: heaviest weights assigned to the category of persons (or biologic unit in the case of the fetus or suckling, as I will discuss in a moment), a somewhat lighter weight to family, still lighter to subculture, community and so on (Fig. 14-2). I do not mean to imply that there can be a formula for computing the worth of research studies in perinatal medicine. But I do suggest that in our plural society, dominant-culture definitions of "risk" and "benefit" should not be applied across-the-board. For example, what is the risk-to-benefit ratio of a proposal to investigate the pharmacologic control of labor and delivery with the drug oxytocin as compared with standard obstetric practice? The purported benefit of this hormone is efficient induction and augmentation of uterine contractions during labor, and the possible risk is a small increase in jaundice among newborn infants leading to a small possibility that treatment of the jaundice will be required by exchange blood transfusion. The risk-to-benefit ratio is very much higher for Jehovah's Witnesses (p 116), I argue, than for others who define the risk of blood transfusion in Earth-bound terms. The grounds for exclusion of Jehovah's Witnesses from such a trial are essentially the same as those for excusing conscientious objectors in conventional warfare. For the question of who

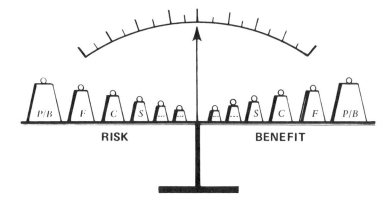

Fig. 14-2. Risks and benefits are appraisals; differential weightings (person/ biologic unit, family, community, subculture . . .) are supplied by different social groups.

should be called upon to participate in clinical studies can only be made "right," Jonas advised, by such authentic identification with the "cause" of the study that it is the subject's as well as the researcher's "cause".

In the hypothetical example which I have chosen, the biologic status of the mother and her about-to-be-delivered infant is straightforward: they are a single biologic entity called the feto-maternal unit. Although this entity changes in physical and physiological detail at the time of birth, the newborn infant continues in an intimate and essential relationship with the mother. The relationship persists for a relatively long period of time. Bostock suggested that man lies somewhere between those mammals whose young walk at birth and the marsupials (like the kangaroo whose young migrate, at a very early stage of fetal life, out of the uterus into a pouch on the mother's abdomen). He argued a thesis which he called "exterior gestation" (comparable to the marsupials): human fetal existence does not end with emergence into the air-breathing world, but with locomotion. To Bostock, human gestation is about 18 months long: 9 months inside and 9 months outside of the uterus. I will not defend this fanciful proposal (although there is a considerable body of evidence which shores up this general idea), but I quote it to make the point that the closeness of this relationship in man should not be underestimated when considering the issues involved in conducting studies during the perinatal period. The archaic term "suckling infants" (which I wish to revive) serves to empha- size the functional facts: mother and child form a symbiotic union—the mother–infant dyad.

In sharp contrast to this biologic view which stresses the oneness of the pair, theologic and legal views emphasize the separateness. Ramsey and Bartholome have written movingly about the fetus and the suckling infant as "persons." And, the language of "rights" has been used to attempt to define their interests as research subjects, particularly in the matter of "informed consent" (who can give permission for the helpless fetus or suckling?). Needless to say, there is very little agreement here. Hauerwas examined some of the arguments and concluded that the issues are well-nigh insoluble in our cultural situation. I agree. Moreover, I believe it has been the arrogant intrusion of religious theories into these secular matters which has served to tangle the issues into a hopeless knot. I do not think the best interests of American families will be served by investing more time and endless arguments in the hope of materializing the mirage of "informed consent." Eisenberg has correctly pointed out that the very justification for a randomized trial is that there is insufficient information to permit a rational, that is, informed choice. In a free society, we reserve the right for any citizen to opt out. But when we respect the privilege to be guided by superstition, astrology, or simple orneriness let us drop the adjective "informed" and speak only of "consent", he concluded. To make the rout complete, the National Commission has abandoned the use of the word consent. In its recommendations, the commission has advised that "permission" of parents or guardians be solicited, to distinguish what a person may do autonomously (consent) from what one may do on behalf of another (grant permission). Additionally, it has been advised that a parent or guardian should be present as much as possible during the conduct of studies in infants. The last recommendation, active participation of parents, deserves special attention. I suspect, for example, that much of the anger and bitterness felt by parents in the years after the RLF incident would have been ameliorated if they had been encouraged to "be present as much as possible" when their infants were in the nursery. If parents had shared the anxieties of nurses and physicians concerning infants in *both* oxygen-management groups in the oxygen trials, there would have been an opportunity for the development of mutual understanding. It is even conceivable to me that the final results of the Cooperative Study in 1954 might have been questioned more by parents than physicians, if they had been active participants.

I propose a plan, *informed surveillance,* which might be used to explore the possibilities of expanding the roles of the principals involved in clinical trials (Fig. 14-3). In addition to the inclusion of parents, the plan places special emphasis on an active role for front-line practicing physicians, for reasons that I will discuss in a moment. We developed a version

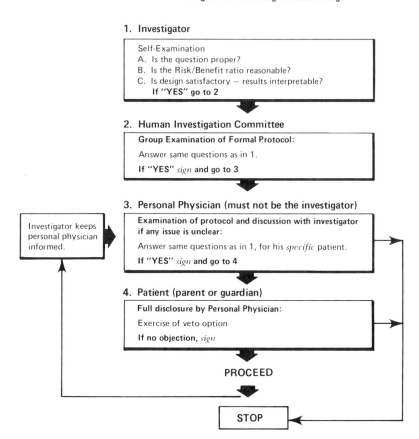

Four Formal Steps in Maintaining Informed Surveillance
in Investigations Involving Human Beings

1. Investigator

Self-Examination
A. Is the question proper?
B. Is the Risk/Benefit ratio reasonable?
C. Is design satisfactory — results interpretable?
If "YES" go to 2

2. Human Investigation Committee

Group Examination of Formal Protocol:

Answer same questions as in 1.

If "YES" *sign* **and go to 3**

3. Personal Physician (must not be the investigator)

Examination of protocol and discussion with investigator if any issue is unclear:

Answer same questions as in 1, for his *specific* patient.

If "YES" *sign* **and go to 4**

Investigator keeps personal physician informed.

4. Patient (parent or guardian)

Full disclosure by Personal Physician:

Exercise of veto option

If no objection, *sign*

PROCEED

STOP

Fig. 14-3.   Flow diagram of a model for informed surveillance in clinical studies.

of this schema for safeguarding studies in premature infants at Babies Hospital in 1953. Our approach was stimulated by a point of view expressed by Guttentag in that year. He noted that the patient–physician relationship may be viewed from two aspects: in one, the physician is an objective, critical investigator; in the other, he is a responsive warm friend who is attentive to the cry for help from his fellow human beings in distress. In present-day highly technical investigation, Guttentag advised that the two facets of the patient–physician relationship be represented by two persons. The "physician-friend" in this division of responsibilities acts to defend the patient's rights and personal welfare when a procedure is proposed by the "physician-investigator." In the model which I propose, there is interaction of three parties (after institutional review and approval of a formal protocol of procedures to be used in a proposed study): (1), the physician-investigator, who is charged with the responsibility of informing the personal physician and answering questions on every detail of the study; (2), the personal physician, who is charged with the responsibility of *attempting* to inform parents about the details of the study and to reply to their questions which may arise before and at all stages of the investigation; and (3), parents, who are asked to give tentative permission for enrollment in the investigation only by indicating that they have *no objection* to proceeding. It has been pointed out that an explanation and an offer of choice simply are not enough to obtain informed consent (to use the abandoned terms for a moment). The quality of consent is not the same when the social distance between doctor and parents is great, as it is when they are more nearly social equals. The veto options of parents and of personal physician should be retained by them at all stages of the investigation. They should not be made to feel any obligation to adhere to the agreement made at the time of enrollment in a clinical trial; "second thoughts" should be respected without coercion.

If veto options are exercised so frequently that a trial is "ruined," the significance of this turn of events should not be overlooked. From a community-oriented perspective, the rates of noncomplicance and defection by parents and personal physician are basic pieces of information. Since the entire *raison d'etre* for *human* experiments lies in the potential for projecting results to the community-at-large, clinical trials must be designed to generate useful information bearing on this fundamental objective. If parents and personal physicians are unable to identify with the goals of the trial and do not perceive themselves as active participants, there is little reason to expect that an outcome of interest to the investigator will be of any public interest.

As I have already indicated, special efforts should be made to enlist the aid and to stimulate the interest of practicing physicians in formal clinical studies. For, it is the practitioner who must translate the results of these efforts into everyday practice. Chalmers has documented some examples of the disturbing effect when physicians feel alienated from research efforts. He examined the extent to which the practice of medicine is a reflection of controlled clinical trials. There was a clear-cut dichotomy between the "usual practice of the community" and the hard-won scientific data. Physicians seemed to be paying no attention to the reports of carefully designed studies. This happened after the 1954 study of RLF; physicians disregarded the results of the massive trial and administered oxygen to premature infants in concentrations below 40 percent in the belief that this was safe (p 51). During the same period another disturbing incident occurred in which pregnant women received DES (Diethylstilbestrol). In the early 1950s this hormone was used to treat early complications of pregnancy, particularly in the hope of preventing miscarriage in women with a past record of habitual fetal loss. At the time of its use, there was no known toxicity. Enthusiastic endorsements were based on the results of seven uncontrolled observational studies, but six investigations found no beneficial effect. All six of the studies which gave negative results used contolled-trial methodology and three of these trials were double-blind (neither physician nor patient knew, in each instance, whether hormone or inactive placebo had been given, and the identification of patients as "treated" or "control" was not disclosed until after the outcomes were recorded). As Chalmers has pointed out, these findings should have been impressive to practicing physicians. The evidence that the estrogenic drug had no effect in preventing miscarriage in any group of patients was quite substantial. Six of seven textbooks of obstetrics came to this conclusion in the 1960s. Despite this, during the period between 1960 and 1970 an average of ca. 100,000 prescriptions for DES per year were written for women who were pregnant. And there was evidence of geographic differences: (1) use of the drug for prenatal care was more "fashionable" in the East and Midwest than in the South and West (3.67 and 2.93 vs 1.94 and 1.68 DES prescriptions per 100 live births), and (2) use of the hormone varied considerably between hospitals located in different areas of the United States (from 1.5 percent of pregnancies in a Boston hospital to zero among 3460 pregnancies in a Baltimore hospital). This was years after evidence from the controlled studies indicated that the treatment had no demonstrable beneficial effect. Beginning in 1972, it was observed that cancer of the vagina was developing in some young women whose mothers had received the hormone while pregnant. The total dimensions of the DES disaster have not yet been determined.

Undoubtedly, many proposals will be made to find a way through the maze of difficulties which complicate use of the experimental method in clinical studies involving the fetus and suckling infant. The National Commission's report serves a useful, but limited, function: it indicates where the *wrong* turns are located. However, I find it hard to believe there will be anything more than token movement until parents, practicing physicians, ethicists, lawyers and legislators insist on the use of scientifically rigorous methodology because of the inherent safety of the approach. Additionally, general acceptance of new treatments in the future may involve governments and voters who demand a slower but better-coordinated advance in this field of activities; a pace that does justice to the processes, functions, and purposes of life. H. Mahler, Director-General of the World Health Organization, has said that objective assessment must go beyond technical considerations. Communities have a right to make value judgments concerning new developments. Mahler advised that critical evaluation of new interventions must entail not only controlled clinical trials, but an additional step: controlled *community* trials on ways of delivering fully assessed technologies to specific communities. The Director-General was referring to the problems which have resulted from the unevaluated use of complex medical technology in underdeveloped countries. But his cautions should be considered in the developed countries as well. For instance, the criticism of the Oxford consumer group (p 110) suggests that even after perinatal intensive care technology has been fully evaluated from a medical point of view, it should not be imposed on a community without a planned trial to evaluate the full social effects of this intervention.

Finally, I propose exploration of a change in experimental strategies based on a different approach to the theory of scientific knowledge: a shift from the validation-of-hypotheses tack to Popper's "refutability" formulation. He observed that science is not a system of certain or well-established statements; nor is it a system which advances toward a state of finality. Since it can never claim to have attained the truth, the method of research should not defend conjectures in order to prove how right we are. And, since a single *definitive* refutation stands out against countless confirmations, Popper advised that we try to overthrow suppositions, using all the logical, mathematical, and technical weapons available. (No matter how many thousands of times that loud noise has been shown to "cure" a solar eclipse, a single test consisting of a few minutes of silence is enough to overturn the theory.) Popper holds that all theories are tentative, never certain: a scientific "truth" is merely a statement which has thus far resisted refutation. Moreover, the requirement that statements should be *capable* of being proven erroneous sets them apart from metaphysical statements which are not refutable by any conceivable event (Galen's claim for his failure-proof remedy is a good example of a metaphysical assertion in medicine, p 128).

Popper's thesis that test-by-refutation has a privileged place (over that of test-by-verification) is not acceptable to some students of the philosophy of science; but I do not wish to become involved in the controversy. The point I wish to make is that his refutation approach has some important practical advantages as a theoretical base for clinical studies; for, in bed-side medicine the temporality and provisional nature of "truth" is taken for granted. Experimental designs to place proposals at maximum risk of invalidation require considerably more planning and ingenuity than are needed to mount corroborative studies. Most importantly, the aim of a severe test is not necessarily the total destruction of each theory, but to obtain information about the limits of its applicability (or safety). For example, at the conclusion of the 1954 Cooperative Study of RLF this statement appeared in the final report: "Limiting the duration [of stay] in oxygen to that deemed necessary to meet frank clinical emergency was shown to be without effect on the survival rate of the premature infant." From the Popperian point of view which I propose, one is obliged to ask: What are the limits of applicability of this assertion?, and, importantly, Was the 1954 test of the long-held fears of oxygen curtailment a *vigorous* test? The answer to the second question is, No. The mortality risk among the infants in the study (all were enrolled after reaching the age of 48 hours) was relatively low when compared with the risk in the first two days of life. The curtailment-of-oxygen-is-safe theory was not tested under con-ditions where it would be placed in maximum jeopardy. As a result, the 1954 declaration of "no significant difference" in mortality (setting aside the semantic problems which surround the phrase, see chapter notes) should be regarded as very provisional, indeed. Popper notes the paradox that the more a theory says, then the more it excludes or forbids, and the greater the opportunities for falsifying it. This relationship between greater content and higher falsifiability is seen in these two assertions:

1. Curtailment of oxygen for premature infants is safe.
2. Curtailment of oxygen for premature infants *under* 48 hours of age is safe.

The content of the second statement is greater than the first: it provides more information. But the second excludes more than the first: it prohibits an acute protective effect confined to the first two days of life. And it has more opportunity to be falsified. This is the essence of Popper's thesis: our knowledge grows by the process of replacing any given assertion with a more risky theory—one less likely to hold up to experiments or tests.

Obviously, a critical test of the effects of oxygen restriction in the first 48 hours of life would have required considerable thought, planning, and care if the disputed issues were to be examined in a responsible manner. And it would have been a very difficult trial to carry out. But the results would have provided some objective evidence concerning a problem which has plagued physicians for almost a quarter of a century. And it goes without saying that the well-being of countless infants would have been protected by the critical approach which seeks to narrow the area of uncertainty. In this regard, the Popperian aim is just the opposite of that in evangelism which seeks to convert and to generalize without limit.

It is relatively easy to make any theory appear credible if we concentrate on collecting confirmatory observations from the world of experience. For example, the initial observations on the success of ACTH, oxygen curtailment, detergent-mist, half-skimmed cow's-milk mixtures, and DES were all supported by repeated confirmatory observations. Only the attempts to put each of these clusters of favorable experiences (like the runs of consecutive "heads" in coin-tossing) to a formal test, a test which risked the possibility that the initial good results would *not* be confirmed, succeeded eventually in narrowing the areas of uncertainty about the proposals. Perhaps the lessons from the past and the implication of Popper's logic will change the emphasis from validation to limits of application in future studies involving children. I sincerely hope so.

Scio (I know), the presumptuous slogan of medicine, should, at long last, be replaced by the modest *Quaero* (I seek). This was fully appreciated by Claude Bernard. In reference to the tentative nature of results obtained after the most painstaking methods to arrive at the "truth," he said,

> There are only partial and provisional truths which are necessary to us as steps on which we rest so as to go on with investigations.

APPENDICES

APPENDIX A

"Causes" of RLF
First Ten Years (1942–1952)

Factors Speculated as the Cause of RLF	Retrospective Correlations ("Passive Observations")	Prospective Clinical Trials (Experimental or Quasi-Experimental)
A. *Parental Factors*		
1. Causes of premature birth		
a. Multiple birth	High frequency in twins Identical (monovular) —twins both usually affected Fraternal twins—one or both affected	
b. Toxemia of pregnancy		
c. Premature separation of the placenta		
d. Placenta previa		
e. Premature rupture of membranes		
2. Maternal infection		

Factors Speculated as the Cause of RLF	Retrospective Correlations ("Passive Observations")	Prospective Clinical Trials (Experimental or Quasi-Experimental)
a. Smallpox vaccination		
b. Mild clinical infections		
c. Subclinical infections		
3. Nausea of pregnancy		
4. Attempted abortion		
5. Diet during pregnancy		
6. Medication during pregnancy		
7. X-ray examination		
8. Onset of labor		
9. Weight gain during pregnancy		
10. Presentation of the infant		
11. Type of delivery		
12. Type of anesthesia and analgesia		
13. Age of parents		
14. Economic status		
15. Place of conception		
16. Place of residence during pregnancy		
17. Parity of mother	First born more frequently affected in one series; first born less frequently affected in another series	
18. Blood type (Rh)		

Factors Speculated as the Cause of RLF	Retrospective Correlations ("Passive Observations")	Prospective Clinical Trials (Experimental or Quasi-Experimental)
status of the mother		
19. Type or condition of the placenta	Placental deformities more frequent in RLF	
20. Uterine bleeding	Bleeding in pregnancy was more frequent in infants who subsequently developed RLF; another series found no association	

B. *Factors Relating To The Infant*
    1. Season
       a. Month of conception
       b. Month of occurrence of RLF

| 2. Sex | RLF more common in males | |
| 3. Malformations | Skin hemangiomas more frequent in RLF | |

    4. Condition of infant at birth
       a. Resuscitation
       b. Cyanosis (or asphyxia)
       c. Chest wall retractions
       d. Jaundice
       e. Diarrhea
       f. Body temperature

Factors Speculated as the Cause of RLF	Retrospective Correlations ("Passive Observations")	Prospective Clinical Trials (Experimental or Quasi-Experimental)
g. Rate of weight gain		
h. Blood pressure (intra-atrial)		
i. Calcium, phosphorus, phosphatase-level in the blood		
j. Red blood cell resistance to break down		
k. General health	Infants with RLF appeared "weaker;" they remained in the incubators longer and received more transfusions and subcutaneous injections of fluid than others who did not develop the disease	
5. Medical management		
a. Prenatal exposure to X-ray		
b. Exposure to light		Five trials of light exposure vs. eyes covered: all failed to implicate light
c. Initial	RLF more frequent in	

Factors Speculated as the Cause of RLF		Retrospective Correlations ("Passive Observations")	Prospective Clinical Trials (Experimental or Quasi-Experimental)
	thirsting and starving	nurseries which withheld feedings for 2 to 3 days after birth	
d.	Milk feeding	High incidence of RLF in some nurseries using cow's milk-mixture	
		No RLF in a large nursery using only cow's milk-mixture	
e.	Blood transfusion	RLF in infants who received early and repeated transfusions; acute RLF frequently progressed following blood transfusion; on the other hand, RLF in many infants who were never transfused	
f.	Vitamin A deficiency	Eye defects in Vitamin A deficient rats resemble RLF	Large doses of Vitamin A did not prevent RLF in a group of premature infants
g.	Use of water-miscible vitamin supplements and iron	Variation in frequency of RLF correlated with use of water-miscible vitamins and iron (Fig. 3-2)	Frequency of RLF unchanged when multivitamins and iron were excluded from diet of a group of premature infants
h.	Vitamin E	Human premature	Prophylactic and

Factors Speculated as the Cause of RLF	Retrospective Correlations ("Passive Observations")	Prospective Clinical Trials (Experimental or Quasi-Experimental)
deficiency	infant has low levels of vitamin E as compared with mature newborns	therapeutic administration of vitamin E (orally) gave conflicting results: some observed decrease in severity of eye damage, others observed no effect
i. Anoxia and oxygen	Sublethal oxygen-lack leads to damage of vascular tissue— (including retinal vessels of rats)	New cases of RLF continued to develop after reduction in oxygen concentration
	Improper use of oxygen (too rapid removal from sup-plemental oxygen) in premature infants followed by progression of acute RLF	Formal prospective trials reported in late 1952 (see Chapt. 4
	Variation in frequency of RLF (Fig. 3-2) correlated with use of oxygen treatment of premature infants	
	Use of high concentrations of oxygen correlated with rise in frequency of RLF	
	No RLF in a large nursery in U.S. and	

Factors Speculated as the Cause of RLF	Retrospective Correlations ("Passive Observations")	Prospective Clinical Trials (Experimental or Quasi-Experimental)
	in a center in England where oxygen was used freely	
j. Infection (viral agent?)		
k. Hemorrhagic tendency of premature infant	Pre-retinal hemorrhages commonly precede RLF	
l. Delayed retinal coaptation (apposition of retina to underlying choroidal layer of the eye)	Half of small premature infants show delay in coaptation of the retina; RLF developed in many of these infants	
m. Miscellaneous speculations: Uncontrolled new-blood-vessel growth in the retina Uveitis (inflammation of iris, ciliary body and choroid) resulting from un-		

Factors Speculated as the Cause of RLF	Retrospective Correlations ("Passive Observations")	Prospective Clinical Trials (Experimental or Quasi-Experimental)
specified noxious agents		
Ocular hyper-tension		
Careless use of substances which in-fluence growth		

APPENDIX B

Cooperative Study of Retrolental Fibroplasia

The Coordination Committee was composed of:

V. Everett Kinsey, Ph.D., Chairman
Kresge Eye Institute, Detroit, Michigan

Richard L. Day, M.D.
Babies Hospital, New York, New York, and later, State University of New York College of Medicine, Brooklyn, New York

Franklin M. Foote, M.D.
National Society for the Prevention of Blindness, New York, New York

F.M. Hemphill, Ph.D.
School of Public Health, University of Michigan, Ann Arbor, Michigan

Arnall Patz, M.D.
Johns Hopkins Hospital, Baltimore, Maryland

Clement A. Smith, M.D.
Boston Lying-In Hospital, Boston, Massachusetts

Harold Tager
U.S. Public Health Service, N.I.H., Bethesda, Maryland

F. Howell Wright, M.D.
Chicago Lying-In Hospital, Chicago, Illinois

Dr. Harry H. Gordon, a leading authority in the care of premature infants, declined an invitation to serve on the planning committee. Moreover, he was unwilling to have the Harriet Lane premature infant nursery at Johns Hopkins Hospital participate in the proposed study because he believed that the existing evidence was "sufficiently suggestive to warrant recommending use of as little oxygen as necessary to raise premature infants." His experience with changing policies of oxygen therapy while he was at Colorado General Hospital in Denver from 1947–1953 (p 41) suggested that restriction of oxygen was not associated with an increase in mortality of premature infants. Dr. Gordon respected the views of others who disagreed with him, but he believed that the proposed study should be undertaken only by those who were unable to accept the available evidence. He remained in touch with the planning committee and contributed suggestions concerning the final protocol of the national trial.

APPENDIX C

Cooperative Study of Retrolental Fibroplasia

The cooperating hospitals were:

Abington Memorial Hospital, Abington, PA
Baltimore City Hospital, Baltimore, MD
Boston Lying-In Hospital, Boston, MA
Cooper Hospital, Camden, NJ
Bob Roberts Memorial Hospital, Chicago, IL
Michael Reese Hospital, Chicago, IL
Cincinnati General Hospital, Cincinnati, OH
Babies and Children's Hospital, Cleveland, OH
Children's Hospital, Columbus, OH
Charity Hospital, New Orleans, LA
Babies Hospital, New York, NY
Bellevue Hospital, New York, NY
New York Hospital, New York, NY
Hospital of the University of Pennsylvania, Philadelphia, PA
Pennsylvania Hospital, Philadelphia, PA
Temple University Hospital, Philadelphia, PA
Elizabeth Steel Magee Hospital, Pittsburgh, PA
Walter Reed Army Hospital, Washington, DC

The study was supported by funds supplied by the National Institute for Neurological Diseases and Blindness, the National Foundation for Eye Research (Boston), and the National Society for the Prevention of Blindness.

APPENDIX D

Randomized Clinical Trials

Sackett has proposed ten methodologic standards for randomized clinical trials:

A. *Criteria for inclusion in the trial*
   Clinical and demographic characteristics of the study population, as well as the fashion in which it was generated, must be stated clearly . . . to determine the ability to generalize the results to other groups of patients in other locations and situations . . .

B. *Random allocation of study patients*
   Allocation of study patients to alternative treatments must be random, preferably by use of random numbers tables . . .

C. *Prognostic stratification*
   The underlying risk of developing, and dying from, the target outcomes must be identified for members of the study populations. If the subgroups in the study vary widely in the risk of target outcomes [e.g. mortality risk in newborn infants with mild to severe respiratory distress syndrome] consideration must be given to stratifying patients with respect to these risk factors before randomization, so that the comparability of the treatment and the control group is insured. In addition, in describing the results of such a trial, the effects of this prognostic stratification on the subsequent clinical outcomes should be described in detail . . .

D. *Description of the therapeutic maneuver*

The nature of the clinical administration and management of . . . therapy must be stated in sufficient detail to permit the reader to replicate the therapeutic program with precision . . .

E. *Co-morbidity*

Because the presence of a second disease may markedly affect both the ability of patients to function and their subsequent survival, the presence of relevant co-morbid conditions must be identified . . . If co-morbidity is known to affect clinical outcomes or survival . . . in a fashion which may rival the magnitude of the anticipated effectiveness of the [therapy under test], this fact should be taken into account in developing a prognostic stratification of patients before randomization.

F. *Compliance*

The extent to which study population members actually follow therapeutic instructions must be determined and described.

G. *Co-intervention*

The performance of additional screening, diagnostic, and therapeutic procedures upon the experimental group must be avoided unless these same procedures are performed with equal vigor upon members of the comparison group . . .

H. *Contamination*

There must be an attempt to minimize external contamination of the comparison group through the inadvertent administration of the same or related therapeutic agents as those received within the trial by the active therapy group . . .

I. *Diagnostic criteria*

The criteria for determining outcomes of interest, including individual causes of death, must be stated in sufficient detail to permit their application elsewhere . . .

J. *Total morbidity reporting*

Mortality from all causes, as well as that due to the target clinical conditions, must be reported.

NOTES AND REFERENCES

Frontispiece

Maimonides (12th-century physician, Judaic scholar, religious savant . . .) is shown here in a detail from Ben Shahn's watercolor entitled "Apotheosis," with the kind permission of the owner, Mr. Jacob Schulman of Gloversville, New York. The aphorism quoted in this drawing is found in the Babylonian Talmud, Tractate Berachoth 4a.

Preface

Peller (1948) coined the term "perinatal" to refer to the period around and including birth. In recent years the adjective has been used to refer to the unity of fetal and newborn medicine. Chain was quoted in Annotation (1975). Lillian Hellman (1976) has pointed to a peculiarly American characteristic:

> We are a people who do not wish to keep much of the past in our heads. It is considered unhealthy in America to remember mistakes, neurotic to think about them, psychotic to dwell upon them.

See Popper (1962) for the advice concerning critical rationalism.

Chapter 1   A New Affliction in Premature Infants

Doctors Clifford and Chandler kindly responded to my request to recall the details of their first encounter with RLF. Mr. James H. Staton, Director of the Boston Hospital for Women, sent photocopies of the 1940 Boston Lying-In Hospital records of the "first" two infants who were discovered to have RLF (Figs. 1-1 and 1-2), on condition that patients' names be omitted in print. History buffs are referred to Spencer (1955) for these censored details. For the original description of RLF see Terry (1942); he reported a large series of patients three years later (see Terry 1945). Krause (1946) described an association between RLF and congenital malformations of the central nervous system, but there is some doubt about the diagnosis of RLF in this series. For the first description of the serial changes of RLF seen with a direct ophthalmoscope see Owens (1948).

Figure 1-3 is a print of the colored plate which appeared in this classic article. The extreme peripheral areas of the curved retina (where the earliest changes of RLF occur) are difficult to visualize with the direct ophthalmoscope. In recent years, the technique of indirect ophthalmoscopy has been used to examine the eyes of young premature infants. With the latter method the observer sees a larger field of view than with the direct ophthalmoscope, though at smaller magnification and the image is inverted. The earliest changes of RLF (see p 192) seen in the terminal portions of the retinal vessels precede those seen with the direct ophthalmoscope. For a description of the changes seen with modern equipment see Figure 9-1. Figure 1-4 is taken from Patz (1957a): copyright American Academy of Pediatrics 1957.

Chapter 2   Evolvement of Care for
Feeble and Prematurely Born Infants

See Harris (1977) for the anthropologic evidence concerning infanticide. Ancient Roman Law (The Fourth Table of the Justinian Code contains the relevant passage) was quoted in Sandars (1876). Tauber (1958) reviewed the history of infanticide in Japan. See McKeown (1976) for the decline of infanticide as a factor in modern population increase. For a description of early English caretaking, see Commentary (1897). The old quatrain, from Sainte-Marther's book "The Art of Nursing and Rearing Children," was quoted in Lipton (1965). Chaussier's experiment was cited by Zuntz (1906). For the use of mother's milk in enemas and baths see Meissner (1838). The Russian incubator was described by Fürst (1887); the French version, shown in Figure 2-1, is in Denucé (1857). See Dunham (1957) for an account of the history of premature infant care. Ballantyne (1902) described the growth of interest in premature infants in England. Budin's book (1900) was the primer for turn-of-the-century physicians who were interested in this subject. Figure 2-2 is taken from Fürst (1887); it was reproduced in my article on incubator-baby side shows (see Silverman 1979) and appears here with permission of the American Academy of Pediatrics (Copyright 1979). The quote from the French Academy appeared in Commentary (1897). See Winckel (1882) for the womb-like device, Figure 2-3, and Hess (1922) for the Colerat citation. The quotes from Budin appeared in his book (1900). I reported the story of incubator-baby side shows (Silverman 1979); Figure 2-4 appears in that article; copyright American Academy of Pediatrics

1979. According to an 1896 article in The Strand Magazine of London, Doctor Alexandre Lion established premature infant exhibits (Oeuvre Maternelle des Couveuses D'Enfants) in a number of cities in France prior to Couney's first show in Berlin. If this account is true, it casts doubt on Couney's story about the origin of the side-show phenomenon.

Chapter 3   The First Decade of RLF

See Owens (1949a) for the Baltimore study, Hess (1934a) for the Chicago experience, and Kinsey (1949) for the U.S. survey. Reese (1949) found an RLF-like condition described by Collins (1925) as "an opaque membrane behind the lens". Between 1925 and 1937 sporadic examples of (probable) RLF occurred under these typically obscure terms: "metastatic retinitis," "extrauterine endophthalmitis and iridocyclitis," "congenital falciform fold," "shrunken fibrous tissue cataract," "congenital connective tissue formation in the vitreous chamber," and "fibrous tissue cataract." Unsworth (1948) cited a description resembling RLF published in 1820. Table 3-1 is from Lowenfeld (1947) and Figure 3-1 is redrawn from his later article (Lowenfeld 1959). The Boston details and Figure 3-2 (redrawn) are taken from Kinsey (1949). For the vitamin E experience in Baltimore see Owens (1949b) and, in Boston, see Kinsey (1951). After a hiatus of more than 20 years this early experience with vitamine E (alpha tocopherol) prophylaxis has suddenly assumed new importance. Beginning in 1974 (see Johnson 1974 and Phelps 1977), re-investigation of a possible protective effect of vitamin E has raised new hopes for this substance which acts as an antioxidant. For observations of spontaneous regression see Owens (1953). In 1943, Terry suggested that the exposure of the incompletely developed eye to light was, possibly, a cause of RLF. The role of light was discussed for nine years by almost all observers, and anecdotal experiences were cited repeatedly. For example, the frequency of occurrence of RLF appeared to increase with the number of examinations of the eyes of infants with the bright light of the ophthalmoscope. However, no one had examined the question by means of a formal trial. Finally, Locke and Reese (1952) covered one eye in each of 22 premature infants in the nursery of Babies Hospital, New York. The occlusive patch was applied within 24 hours after birth and remained in place until the infants were sent home, 22–75 days later. There was no evidence that RLF could be prevented by occluding light to one eye. Both eyes were then patched in 33 small infants; again, the results failed to implicate light.

Chapter 4   The Oxygen Hypothesis

See K. Campbell (1951) for the quote and the Melbourne data in Table 4-2; Crosse (1951) for the Birmingham data in Table 4-1, and Evans (1951) for the comment about a political evil. Ryan (1952) commented on the introduction of an efficient cot in Melbourne. The contrary experience in Oxford was described by Houlton (1951). The oxygen-lack proposal appeared in Szewczyk (1951). The thesis was roughly the same as one proposed earlier by Ingalls (1948 and 1952) who considered RLF to be a type of congenital malformation caused by inadequate oxygenation before birth or at delivery. Ingalls induced ocular malformations by exposure of pregnant mice to low-oxygen environments, but the changes produced in the developing eyes were not accepted by all critics as typical of RLF. The use of supplemental oxygen to "treat" early RLF was reported by Szewczyk (1952). For the New Orleans report see Exline (1951). The actual concentration of oxygen in the incubators of the New Orleans nursery was not measured. The convective-type incubators used there were of a primitive design. In retrospect, there is reason to suspect that open louvres in these incubators prevented accumulation of significant amounts of supplemental oxygen. For the Paris report and Table 4-3 see Lelong (1952). In a letter to me, Doctor Patz related his conversation with Hoeck, the response to his application, and the nurses reactions. A description of his initial trial, Table 4-4, and the concluding statement appear in Patz (1952).

Chapter 5   The Eye and Oxygen

The embryonic development of the eye was described in Mann (1928). The hyaloid artery forms the fetal intraocular blood system. It arises from the ophthalmic branch of the internal carotid artery, enters the embryonic eye and courses through the vitreous to the posterior surface of the lens. There it breaks up into capillaries which form a network around the lens (the tunica vasculosa lentis). During the sixth month, all vessels of the tunic atrophy, except the hyaloid artery trunk. In the seventh month of gestation, the hyaloid artery shrinks; about the time of birth the artery has disappeared and the permanent retinal circulation is established. Michaelson (1948 and 1954) described the development of *patent* vessels. (His injection method of study revealed only the vessels which had formed a channel, not the cellular events which preceded this stage of development.) Later it was demonstrated (by means of retinal digest and special staining techniques) that the retinal vessels do not develop by a process of budding from the hyaloid artery system, but by preliminary invasion of primitive mesenchymal cells which first appear in the vicinity of the hyaloid artery (see Ashton 1970). The mesenchymal cells differentiate and form a capillary network. According to the present concept, the retinal arteries and veins arise *from* the capillaries (not the reverse as previously supposed). For a present-day description of the "timetable" of retinal vessel growth see Cogan (1963). Ashton (1970) notes that the current concept concerning perivascular capillary-free zones in the retina is different from that put forth by Michaelson. These clear areas appear to develop through capillary retraction rather than by inhibition of capillary growth. Nonetheless, the fact that the zones can be narrowed and widened by lowering and raising ambient oxygen concentration supports the earlier view that oxygen is "antivasculogenic". See F.W. Campbell (1951) for the low-oxygen observations in rats; also Ingalls (1952). High-oxygen effects in mice were described by Gyllensten (1952); salt and water effects in kittens were noted by Hepner (1952). For the clearest report of the oxygen effect see Ashton (1953, 1954 and 1966). Vaso-obliteration in the kitten began in less than 12 hours of exposure to high oxygen and was complete by 36 hours. The obliterative effect was directly related to the duration of exposure in short periods (12, 24 and 36 hours), but was not conclusively shown in studies of longer periods of exposure. Vasoconstriction produced by oxygen exposure was reversible, but total vaso-obliteration, once induced, remained unaltered. Later studies, using a trypsin-digest method to study the capillaries of the retina, indicated that vaso-obliteration begins with capillary closure after about 6 hours' exposure to hyperoxia. This is soon followed by degenerative changes in the cells of the developing vessels. The pathologic changes of blood vessels in human eyes was described by Reese (1951). Figures 5-1 and 5-2 are redrawn from illustrations in Scientific American (Silverman 1977). In a later study, Ashton (1965) found that the proliferative phase was the result of capillary obliteration and not a specific effect related to hyperoxia. When the newborn kitten's retinal vessels were occluded by glass beads, proliferation of vessels into the vitreous occurred (exactly as found after obliteration produced by oxygen exposure). Other animal studies were described by Patz (1953 and 1957a).

Chapter 6   The National
Cooperative Study

There is no reliable accounting of the RLF epidemic. Dependable statistics on blindness in infants were (and continue to be) lacking in the United States. The estimate, "10,000 RLF blind," is an educated guess based on a review of the available, but incomplete, reports from the U.S. and abroad. The details of the Cooperative Study were recorded in the preliminary report (Kinsey 1955) and final report (Kinsey 1956a). It was estimated that about 750 infants would be available for study in the cooperating hospitals in one year. This fixed sample size determined the calculations of the practical limits of the trial. The two outcomes-of-interest, RLF and survival, presented different time problems: the presence or absence of RLF could not be established until each infant was followed for at least three months, but the observation period for survival was arbitrarily set at 40 days. In order to minimize the number of infants exposed to each of the two risks, a complex strategy was devised. Two rates of RLF-incidence were postulated:

"Routine (unrestricted) oxygen"	10–20%
"Curtailed oxygen"	2%

At these rates, a calculated minimum of 50 infants would need to be enrolled in the "routine (unrestricted) oxygen" group in order to obtain results which could be distinguished from chance fluctuation (confidence level of 0.01 percent). It was also assumed that 18 patients would be lost because of death or lack of follow-up. Thus, the number 68 (50 plus 18) was determined for the size of the routine oxygen group. A. Bradford Hill (see p 133) suggested that one infant be assigned to the routine oxygen group for each two infants in the curtailed oxygen group during the first three months of study. This procedure was expected to permit an early-as-possible check of the pretrial postulates concerning the RLF incidence rates in the two groups. If the difference in rates was found to be less than expected, more infants would be assigned to routine oxygen throughout the remainder of the year. The design considerations with respect to survival were different. Here it was expected that week-by-week monitoring of mortality rates in the two groups would quickly disclose a gross disadvantage to infants allotted to "curtailed oxygen" and permit an adjustment of the ratios of infants assigned to the two groups. "Routine (unrestricted) oxygen" was defined as oxygen (concentration over 50 percent) for 28 days. Return to an air environment at or after 28 days by reducing the flow rate of oxygen by one-third over each of three successive days. This regimen was common in the care of small premature infants in 1953. In "curtailed oxygen," supplemental oxygen was administered only if, in the pediatrician's opinion, the clinical condition of the infant demanded it. Concentration not to exceed 50 percent. The concentration of oxygen in incubators was measured three times a day with a paramagnetic analyzer

(Beckman Instruments, Inc.). Birthweight differences, within each set of three, were minimized by allottment within three birthweight categories: ≤1.0 kg (<2 lb 4 oz), 1.0–1.25 kg (>2 lb 5 oz – 2 lb 12 oz), and >1.25 – 1.5 kg (>2 lb 12 oz – 3 lb 5 oz). The New York City Health Department memorandum was entitled, "Recommendations to Hospitals with Materni- ty and Newborn Services." It was signed by Jean Pakter, M.D., Chief of the Maternity and Newborn Division, Department of Health, New York City. The relevant passage from the minutes of the Pediatric Advisory Committee meeting of March 18, 1954 read as follows:

> The meeting opened at 4 P.M. with a brief presentation by Dr. Pakter on the problem of oxygen concentration in relation to retrolental fibroplasia in premature infants. After some discussion by the Committee a motion was made and passed that a recommendation be sent to all hospitals with maternity and newborn services that oxygen should be administered to premature infants only as necessary and then only in concentrations under 40% unless respiratory embarrassment is present. An explanatory statement as to why this recommendation is being made is to be incorporated in the recommendation.

There was no explanation for the fact that the caveat—"unless respiratory embarrassment is present"—which appeared in the minutes, was not re- peated in the circulated recommendation. For the Bellevue results see Lanman (1954). The mortality data in the Bellevue study were recently reexamined (Day 1979):

	Lived	Died	Total	Deaths (%)
High Oxygen	36	9	45	20
Low Oxygen	28	12	40	30

Day and his collaborators noted that the 50 percent increase in mortality *observed* in low oxygen would be expected to occur by chance in about 1 out of 5 repeated trials of this size $(P = 0.21)$. Another way to examine the result of the 1954 Bellevue study is to ask the question: What were the chances of the study being able to declare a 50-percent increase in death rate as significant? The reviewers computed that only 1 out of 8 trials involving 45 babies in one group and 40 in the contrasting group would be expected to detect that a true increase in death rate of 50 percent had taken place. To increase the likelihood of detecting such an important discrepancy in death rate to 8 chances out of 10, it would be necessary to include 313 patients in each of the study groups—a total study enrollment of 626 babies! For the Philadelphia trial see Bedrossian (1954); the Colorado General Hospital experience was summarized by Gordon (1954a). The initial period of the Cooperative Study was focused on the survival issue. The experience in this three-month period was not disclosed until the trial was completed. The results appeared to confirm the favorable impression gained by week-to-week monitoring of short-term outcome in the two oxygen treatment groups:

$$\text{Routine (unrestricted) oxygen} \quad : \quad \frac{15}{68} = 22\% \text{ succumbed}^*$$
$$\text{(July–Dec.)}$$

$$\text{Curtailed oxygen} \quad : \quad \frac{36}{144} = 25\% \text{ succumbed}^*$$
$$\text{(July–Dec.)}$$

All infants were then assigned to curtailed oxygen for the remaining nine months of the study. The results for the final period continued to be reassuring:

$$\text{Curtailed oxygen} \quad : \quad \frac{115}{574} = 20\% \text{ succumbed}^*$$
$$\text{(Oct.–June)}$$

A disturbing rumor about this carefully considered design has been circulated in the years since the trial. Unfortunately, the myth was recorded in 1976 (James 1976):

> Early in the course of the Cooperative Study, it was learned that RLF could be produced experimentally in newborn animals by administering oxygen . . . It was immediately decided that no additional infants should be placed in the routine or "control" group (unrestricted oxygen) and all infnats enrolled after the first three months of study received "curtailed oxygen" therapy.

This statement is untrue, but it has fueled the fires of controversy about the study. The results presented in Table 6-1 appeared in the final report (Kinsey 1956a. The unexpected associations were found by "dredging" the data collected in the Cooperative Study (post eventum). Since no further controlled clinical trials testing oxygen treatment of human infants have been conducted, the associations have not undergone a proper challenge; they must be viewed with these reservations. In kittens (unlike the results in the Cooperative Study) Ashton's group found a relationship

*From enrollment at *age 48 hours* to age 40 days

between concentration of oxygen and *vascular* changes. The severity of the vaso-obliterative effect of oxygen rose with increasing concentration of the gas; concentrations below 35 percent, even after 21 days of continuous exposure, had no effect on the retinal vessels of newborn kittens. The relationship of these observations (vascular changes in a small number of experimental animals) to contrary evidence concerning cicatricial RLF in observations made on a large number of premature infants (p. 000) is unknown. Controlled studies in mice demonstrated that gradual withdrawal does not prevent vascular changes in that species. On the contrary, both the severity and frequency increased in mice when there was additional oxygen exposure during slow reduction of supplemental oxygen (Gyllensten 1956 and Patz 1957b). The rise and fall of RLF in New York State was reported by Yankauer (1956a).

Chapter 7   Oxygen Treatment
Practices in Premature Infants

Early recommendations were given by Budin (1900), Ylppö (1917), Hess (1922) and Bakwin (1923). Figure 7-1 is taken from Hess (1934a); reproduced with permission of the publisher, copyright The University of Chicago Press, 1934. The experience summarized in Table 7-1 appeared in Hess (1934b). See Wilson (1942) for the observations made in Detroit (depicted in Fig. 7-2). Nineteen years earlier Bakwin (1923) had quoted authorities who considered periodic breathing to be due to oxygen lack; Cheyne-Stokes breathing in adults was abolished by giving oxygen. Bakwin observed that when oxygen was administered to *cyanosed* premature infants, color improved and respirations became more regular. See Smith (1942) for the concept of "subcyanotic anoxia." In the mid-1930s, Chapple conceived the idea of building an incubator that would (1) protect premature infants from exposure to air-borne micro-organisms, and (2) maintain stable surrounding conditions of temperature, humidity and oxygen. He concluded that "the infant would have to be kept in an incubator which did not need to be opened to care for them." Access to the infant was accomplished through balloon cloth sleeves. The cabinet was ventilated by fresh air "drawn from out of doors" (filtered, heated and humidifed before it was blown into the closed infant compartment). Oxygen was introduced through a tube connected to a mask or funnel inside of the box. The first experimental model was installed in November 1937 at the Children's Hospital of Philadelphia (see Chapple 1938). Approximately 35 incubators of this design were used exploratively, in Abington, Baltimore, Boston, Germantown, New Haven and New York City (Brooklyn) in the years before World War II. A commercially marketed version of the individually ventilated Chapple-type incubator became available in the late 1940s. Air-Shields, Inc. made the drawings of the incubator (Fig. 7-3) and the air-oxygen intake (Fig. 7-4). See Yankauer (1955) for the New York State memorandum. See Lanman (1955) for the 40-percent oxygen quote, Guy (1956) for the paper indicating the possibility of eliminating RLF. See Kinsey (1956b) for the letter cautioning against the emphasis on 40 percent oxygen, Gordon (1957) for the letter pointing out the defect in the Cooperative Study. The decision to limit enrollees in the Cooperative Study to those infants who survived 48-hours was reached with full appreciation of the fact that most of the deaths related to premature birth occur in the first two days of life. These early deaths, it was argued, would not help answer the question of oxygen damage to the developing retinal vessels. This strategy also took into account the fact that no restriction on oxygen administration in the first two critical days would be more acceptable to many nurses who were resistant to a proposed policy of oxygen restriction. Gordon did not indicate in his letter the magnitude of the risk of dying in the first 48 hours of life in 1953-54 among infants weighing $\leq$ 1.5 kg at birth. This can be appreciated from the following statement, which appeared in the final report of the Cooperative Study (Kinsey 1956a):

786 survived 48 hours* and were enrolled in the study . . . there were 634 additional premature infants in this birthweight category born in or brought to these hospital nurseries during this [one-year] period. All of these were reported to have died before 48 hours.

Chapter 8   Consequences of
Oxygen Restriction

The totals in Figure 8-1 are based on articles listed in Quarterly Cumulative Index 1942-56, Current List of Medical Literature 1957-59, and Cumulative Index Medicus 1960-62. See Editorial (1974) for a summary of RLF unrelated to supplemental oxygen. The rare examples of *congenital* RLF observed since Reese and Blodi's original description in 1951 were, and remain, a puzzle; they are often regarded as variants of oxygen-induced RLF and difficult to classify. On the other hand, Ashton's demonstration (1965) that vasoproliferative changes occur irrespective of the cause of obliteration of the developing retinal vessels makes it fairly

*Among the enrollees, 166 died before age 40 days.

easy to accept these congenital instances as "true" RLF. The infant described in 1951 had typical microscopic changes of RLF. Birthweight was 1.95 kg, and he was thought to be full-term. The baby died soon after birth, and, in addition to RLF, had anencephaly. A later example of congenital RFL was associated with hydrocephalus. See Avery (1960) for the Johns Hopkins evidence (summarized in Table 8-1) and the concluding quote. In 1959 (see Silverman 1961), I reviewed the annual occurrence of hyaline membrane disease at Babies Hospital from 1950 through 1957 (the years before and after oxygen restriction). Crude annual mortality rate and proportion of dead infants examined at autopsy did not vary appreciably from year to year, and annual fluctuations in "incidence" of hyaline membrane disease exhibited no significant trend-change. However, these uncontrolled retrospective observations suffered from the same interpretive limitations as those at Johns Hopkins Hospital. See McDonald (1962) for the English follow-up results, the data shown in Fig. 8-2 and the quote. The Clark polarographic oxygen measuring device was first described in 1956 (Clark 1956). When this instrument became generally available in the early 1960s it was possible to measure oxygen tension of the blood quickly and reliably. To demonstrate that it was oxygen in blood (not in the air surrounding the eye) Ashton (1964) performed these experiments: pure oxygen passed through a cup over one eye of a newborn kitten for three days produced no retinal vessel changes; pure oxygen beathed by kittens for the same period resulted in typical retinal abnormalities. The low tensions of oxygen in arterial blood drawn from the lower aorta of infants with respiratory distress was largely due to shunting of blood from the right to left sides of the heart through fetal channels (see Strang 1961). This blood is unoxygenated because it is diverted to the aorta before there is any contact with the lungs. See Warley (1962) for the Oxford studies. See Silverman (1968) for a report of the 1967 meeting concerning oxygen and RLF.

Chapter 9   The Determinative Era of
Oxygen Treatment

The pure oxygen breathing test (Table 9-1) is described in Roberton (1968). The National Society's hospital survey was conducted by Mrs. E.M. Hatfield (see Silverman 1969). The distribution of grades of RLF found in the survey (1,117 hospitals which delivered 1000 or more infants each year) was as follows:

Vascular RLF	18
Cicatricial RLF	14
Stage not reported	1
Total	33

From past experience (Chapter 3) it was expected that in 3 out of 4 infants who develop RLF the blood vessel changes would not go on to scarring (cicatricial stage). Since the survey indicated that about half ended in the vascular stage, I interpreted this to indicate that many infants with early RLF were not examined. In 1976 (Akeson 1976), the Variety Blind Babies Foundation and the Educational Services for Preschool Blind Children were (between them) serving 63 preschool children throughout the State of California. The birth dates of these children were distributed as follows:

1970 — 4;
1971 — 8;
1972 — 12;
1973 — 12;
1974 — 17;
1975 — 10.

The 1969 Cooperative Study involved Columbia, Johns Hopkins, McGill, Vanderbilt and Washington (Seattle) Universities. The study was co-directed by Doctors Arnall Patz and V. Everett Kinsey. The results of this study were published in 1977 (Kinsey 1977). Doctor John T. Flynn kindly supplied the photographs in Fig. 9-1. Flynn's group (Kushner 1977 and Flynn 1977) has postulated that precursors of the normally developing capillary network of the retina (chords and sheets of mesenchymal tissue which grow out from the optic disc just ahead of vessels) are involved in development of the distinctive "silver line" structure in early RLF. According to this hypothesis, hyperoxia obliterates newly formed capillaries, particularly in the region just behind the advancing border of mesenchyme. The mesenchyme ceases to migrate and piles up as a shelf of tissue. Arteries and veins empty into the structure (by a few remaining bridges of blood vessels) to begin formation of a vascular shunt. In most instances regression occurs when buds of new vessels arise from the advancing edge of the shunt; vascularization proceeds leading, eventually, to near-normal retinal blood supply and a normally functioning eye. Persistence and progression of the abnormal changes, in a minority of instances (Flynn estimates ca. 15 percent), leads to the familiar damaging lesions of cicatricial RLF. See also Baum (1971b), Mushin (1974) and Kingham (1977) for present-day observations of the early changes of RLF by photography, fluorescein angiography and indirect ophthalmoscopy. See Baum (1971a) for the residual changes of tortuosity which resemble the findings in the proliferative phase of RLF (esp. hairpin bends in the retinal arteries as in Fig. 9-2, which was kindly supplied by Doctor Baum). Other associations suggested that these minor changes were those of aborted RLF:

a.   The temporal branches of retinal arteries were more often involved than the nasal segments (a well-known finding in acute vascular RLF).

b.   Arterial tortuosity was associated with low gestational age, and was significantly less evident in those persons known to have had a more advanced gestational age than expected from their birth weight. It is reasonable to presume that the retinal vessels were more mature at birth in this group of individuals than in others of similar birth weight with appropriate gestational age.

c.   In another set of observations the frequently occurring vascular changes seen by photography and fluorescein angiography were more common in multiple births (another well-known RLF association).

No definite pattern of refractive error was found in the eyes of the 35 persons with only arterial tortuosity of retinal vessels. Scarring (incomplete) RLF in 10 people was associated with myopia; curvature of the cornea was normal in these eyes. The invention of a device for continuous monitoring of the transcutaneous oxygen by means of a skin electrode (see R. Huch 1973 and A. Huch 1979) has had the effect of perpetuating the preoccupation with the role of oxygen in RLF. In addition to technical questions concerning this approach (e.g. which, if any, skin sites provide the best estimate of the state of oxygenation of the retina?) there remains the unanswered problem of RLF which occurs at "normal" arterial tensions. See Johnson (1974) and Phelps (1977) for vitamin E studies. See Aranda (1975) for observations concerning blood transfusions and RLF. See Cross (1973) for the calculations concerning the cost of preventing RLF and Bolton (1974) for the data shown in Fig. 9-4. Deaths on the day of birth were considered to be related to the policy of uncritical oxygen restriction. The hypothesis predicted that the deviation from a continuous fall in mortality would be trivial in babies born at term (normal birthweight) in whom respiratory troubles are relatively infrequent. This was borne out in the experience in New York State examined by Bolton (1974). There were numerous confounding influences during the years of rising day-of-birth deaths (e.g. influenza epidemics in the 1950s, large number of drug-related deaths caused by sulfisoxazole and chloramphenicol—see Chapter

10—during the same period) and many major changes in neonatal care during the time of, and subsequent to, the fall in day-of-birth deaths. The conclusion of the 1953-54 Cooperative Study concerning the non-relationship between oxygen concentration and RLF (p 41) was based on after-the-fact analyses. A formal strategy in which infants were allocated in random order to prescribed exposure to specific concentrations of oxygen below 50 percent was not incorporated into the 1953-54 investigation. Recently, the St. Louis Society for the Blind honored Doctor Szewczyk for his work on the RLF problem. He was quoted (Szewczyk 1977) as follows:

> . . . since the policy of gradual withdrawal from high oxygen concentration was instituted in 1951 only three out of more than 4800 babies born at the hospital have suffered blindness from RLF, although others have suffered a lesser degree of vision impairment.

See Hatfield (1975) for the prevalence data depicted in Fig. 9-5 (the *existing* number of affected children per 100,000 pupils). A.G. Jenkins, Director of the Orientation Center for the Blind, Albany, California, told me of the performance of the RLF-blinded man. Doctor Berthold Lowenfeld, former Director of the California School for the Blind, recently recalled his impressions concerning the behavior of RLF-blinded children when they arrived at his school in the 1950s. His experience in teaching blind children goes back to Vienna at the turn of the century when syphilis, gonorrhea and severe bacterial infections accounted for most of the blindness in young children. He said

> . . . then, early in the century, we knew children were damaged; those children showed mental retardation, inability to get along with others, quite out of the way, but here we had RLF children who showed behavior with which we were not familiar . . . and, of course, the name "autism" was tagged on these youngsters, and a good deal of observation was done; but no conclusive evidence has been submitted . . .

Elonen (1964) noted that the irregular pattern of development in blind children frequently leads to a mistaken diagnosis of mental retardation. She listed a number of "pseudo-conditions" in blind children and the circumstances which contribute to these manifestations:

Pseudo-condition	*Contributing Circumstances*
a. Chewing difficulties	Prolonged bottle feeding, late introduction of solids
b. Passivity/dependence	Waited on (carried, fed, dressed, guided . . .)
c. Spatial disorientation	Restricted exploration

d.	Speech–language	Bombarded with sound, over-response to nonverbal signals (family), absent facial-gesture signals
e.	Conceptualization	Lack of visual challenges (scenes) and clues (depth, size, color)
f.	Loneliness/lone-ism	Limited experience with other children
g.	Dearth of pleasant fantasy	Increased experience with hospitals, surgery, falls, accidents and separations
h.	Auto-erotic habits	Seductive behavior of adults

See also Chase (1972) and Fraiberg (1977) for descriptions of the behavior of RLF-blinded children. At the time when plans for the 1953-54 Cooperative Study were discussed, the need for long-term followup of participants was brought up. Unfortunately, the opportunity for systematic observations, as I pointed out earlier, was missed. In 1976, federal support was requested to examine a cohort of RLF-blind young adults and compare their neurologic status (esp. spatial orientation) with controls (other congenitally blind and a group of sighted ex-prematures). The proposal was rejected by reviewers with the statement, ". . . much of the information sought by the study is mainly of historical value." Patz (1955) reported that extensive examination of all organs in newborn mice, rats and kittens exposed to prolonged high concentrations of oxygen failed to reveal changes in any tissues except the eye and occasionally the lung. On the other hand, Gyllensten (1959) found retarded development of capillaries in the brain of young mice reared in high-oxygen environments. In rats, residual brain damage has been seen only after exposure to very high oxygen tension (4–5 atmospheres). See also Balentine (1966) for oxygen effects on the brain of rats. See Feeney (1976) and Dormandy (1978) for a discussion of the biochemical mechanism of oxygen toxicity.

Chapter 10   Medical Inflation

A somewhat modified version of this chapter appears in Perspectives in Biology and Medicine, Summer 1980. See Wallace (1950) and Silverman (1961) for demographic information on the incidence of prematurity. Yankauer (1956b) described the New York–Cornell institutes. Doctor Chapple recalled that Chestnut Hill Hospital near Philadelphia was among the first institutions to express an interest in his new incubator (after the initial experimental period, see p 189). He delivered a hand-built model to the hospital in a borrowed pick-up truck in the summer of 1938. A 2 lb 10 oz infant was reared in the device without any swaddling clothes. He and Doctor Aims C. McGuiness (the infant's pediatrician) spent every spare moment staring at the baby—the first naked premature infant anyone had observed for an extended period of time. Toward the end of the first year of use of the new incubator, Doctor Chapple became aware that the nurses were resisting the practice of caring for nude infants. They seemed ill at ease when a naked boy suddenly sprayed conspicuously. A compromise was struck to preserve modesty: diapers! See Silverman (1961) for the development of premature centers and Taylor (1948) for a report of the Colorado program. See Pakter (1954) for the history of the New York City program for premature infant centers. Some indication of the immediate (hospital) cost for premature infant care in the 1970s is given in a report by Pomerance (1978): the average daily cost for infants weighing less than 1 kg at birth was $534/day/infant in September 1976 (by November 1977 this rate had increased by 31 percent). Murphy (1951) described North Carolina developments. See Bloxom (1950) and Reichelderfer (1956) for the "air-lock" experience. See Ravenel (1953), Silverman (1955) and Briggs (1955) for the detergent-mist details; and Silverman (1956a) for further observations on water-mist. See Smith (1949 and 1957) for observations of effects of delaying feedings. See Ylppö (1954-55) for the European arguments and Gleiss (1955) for the German evidence against the fasting practice. See Drillien (1961) and D.P. Davies (1978) for the observations on brain damage (esp. spastic diplegia) in relation to first-feed practices. For the New York studies on fat absorption and its implications, see Gordon (1941). See Menkes (1966) for the report of a follow-up study of transient tyrosinemia in the newborn period. The taurine hypothesis was advanced by Gaull (1977). See Clifford (1950) for the prophylaxis, and Silverman (1956b) for the sulfisoxazole experience. See Alexander (1957) and Burns (1959) for the chloramphenicol observations. See Katz (1972) and Insight Team (1979) for the details concerning thalidomide. The "therapeutic programs which evolve . . ." quote appeared in a letter written to me by Doctor William H. Tooley on May 9, 1972. The "Proclaimed Therapies" noted in Table 10-2 were widely applied long before formal evaluation was carried out. In most instances, the practices faded away (became "unfashionable") without a formal test. See Agerty (1952) for the results of a trial of testosterone treatment which failed to show any significant influence on weight gain. Years after the attempts to stimulate the growth of premature infants with this powerful hormone were abandoned, some disturbing animal studies came to light; early treatment with male sex hormone had an effect on sexual-orientation behavior at maturity. Follow-up studies of the testosterone-treated babies were never undertaken. A double-blind controlled study of the effects of thyroid hormone (see Stevenson 1953) indicated that this treatment was without recognizable benefit and was sometimes harmful (diarrhea and increased pulse rate were observed in treated infants). The DES experience is described on p 158. Masculinization of the female fetus may follow administration of progestins (especially when given prior to the 13th week of pregnancy—see Grumbach 1959). See Allen (1957) for an account of the use of exchange transfusion in the management of erythroblastosis fetalis. The exact criteria for use of this technique to treat jaundice caused by other mechanisms has been debated for years. The use of oxygen for periodic breathing is discussed on p 46. See note above for the issues in initial thirsting and starving. Meyer (1956) described jaundice and kernicterus caused by synthetic vitamin K. See note above for the low-fat–high-protein feeding experience, the sulfisoxazole episode and the chloramphenicol incident. The stomach of newborn infants was suctioned at birth in the hope that this would prevent the development of respiratory difficulty. Several trials were conducted (see Westin 1958); none were able to demonstrate a beneficial effect. Traction on the sternum to stabilize the soft chest wall of infants with respiratory difficulty was proposed, used half-heartedly, but never evaluated formally (see Townsend 1956). For the epsom-salts see note below. A rocking device (see Millen 1955) to prevent respiratory problems was used for several years; there was no convincing evidence that the apparatus was effective. The Alevaire and water-mist reports are noted above. See Chu (1967) for the experience indicating that administration of acetylcholine may be beneficial to infants with respiratory distress syndrome. The authors advised that their uncontrolled study results should not be accepted until a convincing test was carried out using proper experimental design (and they warned that the swiftly acting, dangerous drug should be administered with great caution). Nonetheless, the agent was used by others, but the purported beneficial effects on survival were never put to a critical test by the original observers (nor by anyone else). See Donald (1954) for an early description of the use of a respirator to support premature infants. Belenky (1978) discussed the weakness of the evidence to support the widely used and accepted measure of constant positive airway pressure. See Vengusamy (1969) for results of a controlled clinical trial which demonstrated a higher mortality with gastrostomy than with routine oral feedings in groups of very small infants (birthweights 0.75– 1.25 kg = 1 lb 10 oz – 2 lb 12 oz). See Miller (1957) for the animal experiments on the use of cold in resuscitation. Ice-water resuscitation was used in delivery rooms for years; it was slowly abandoned after it was shown that the newborn infant makes a metabolic response to cold exposure. Sodium bicarbonate injections were used extensively to treat early acidemia in the hope that this would prevent hyaline membrane disease; Hobel (1972) was unable to confirm these hopes from the results of a well-planned controlled trial involving 90 babies. See Finberg (1967) for the evidence which suggests that rapid injections of alkali are dangerous. See p 105 for the relation of temperature to survival. See Powell (1973) for the description of the dangers of hexachlorophene bathing. See Speck (1975) for the possibility of damage to chromosomal material from exposure to phototherapy. The list of treatments in Table 10-2 is not complete; see Moore (1976) for futher misadventures which followed those presented in this table. The "I am disturbed at . . . ." quote appeared in a discussion of the paper by Clifford (1950). See Coleman (1957) for the sociologic study. Soon after the New York Times article announced the effect of epsom-salt enemas, a query was received by the editor of *Pediatrics*. The writer (see Van Gelder 1965) expressed concern about the safety of dehydrating enemas for desperately ill infants and he was disturbed by the fact that physicians were under considerable pressure to use the treatment as the result of the wide publicity. He requested guidance from the journal (the official organ of te American Academy of Pediatrics). The plea was sent to the originator of the new approach; when a reply was received both letters were printed in the February, 1965 issue. The innovator repeated his rationale (which was explained in full in a later report—see Stowens 1965) and his letter of reply ended with these words, "I am happy to be able to report that since the appearance of the newspaper and magazine stories, numerous physicians around the country, who have not shared Doctor Van Gelder's querulousness or inability to reach independent conclusions, have reported to me of their successes with this form of therapy." See Andrews (1965) for the effects of magnesium sulfate in newborn lambs, and Outerbridge (1973) for the report of a death following an epsom-salt enema treatment. The incredible Laetrile situation is described in Sounding Board (1978). Indeed, the emotion surrounding Laetrile threatens the legislative safeguards erected after the thalidomide incident (see p 83). See Naftulin (1973) for the "Doctor Fox" phenomenon.

Chapter 11   The Price of Progress

The data in Table 11-1 were calculated from information provided by Richard W. Turlington, Information Officer, Division of Research Grants, N.I.H., and from U.S. Bureau of the Census (1975). Table 11-2 was prepared from listings in Quarterly Cumulative Index Medicus 1950 and

1955 and Index Medicus 1960. See Price (1961 and 1963) for analysis of the growth of science. The Russian scientist's remark is apocryphal. See Pakter (1974) for the birth rate/infant mortality experience in New York City, and Lee (1976) for the Bronx Municipal Center analysis. See Morris (1975) for evaluation of causes of decline in infant mortality in the U.S. Intermediate infant mortality was defined as a rate equal to the observed overall infant mortality plus or minus 10 percent, using data from a 1960 U.S. Live Birth Cohort Study to define the high-risk and low-risk maternal-age/total-birth-order cells shown in Fig. 11-1. The 1960s infant mortality rates for each age/total-birth-order cell were applied to the age/total-birth-order distributions of births for each of the succeeding years. This calculation provided the estimated number of deaths in each cell for these years under an assumption of constant age/total-birth-order mortality rates within each cell. The sum of the estimated deaths for each year was then compared with the actual number of deaths to measure the contribution of changing age–parity distributions. See Hinds (1974) for the relation between infant mortality and numbers of health-care workers, and St. Leger (1978) for the correlation with "doctors available" (Fig. 11-2 is redrawn from this report). See Neligan (1974) for the Newcastle study. The U.S. studies were reported by Broman (1975), Werner (1967) and Jordan (1970). See Drillien (1967) for the Edinburgh results. The University College Hospital results and subsequent English reports are summarized by P.A. Davies (1976). See McCormick (1977) for the eye survey results. See Sameroff (1975) for the "continuum of caretaking casualty" thesis, Werner (1971) for outcomes at ten years of age in 1000 live births, and Baum (1977) for his comments on families. Also see Stratton (in Chard 1977) for a review of the evidence concerning perinatal circumstances and later development. See Jonsen (1975) for Doctor Nader's comments.

Chapter 12   Progress in a Groove

See Chard (1977) for criticism of perinatal medicine. See Whitehead (1925) for his quote. See Silverman (1958) for the temperature results. See MacMahon (1977) for U.S. cause-of-death data and life-expectancy trends; Wegman (1977) for recent infant mortality. See Harris (1977) for a discussion of female infanticide, and Birdsell quoted by Harris. Figures 12-1 and 12-2 are redrawn from Shapiro (1968). See Grove (1968) and National Center for Health Statistics (1977) for the data in Table 12-1. McKeown (1976) examined the causes of modern population rise. See Erbe (1977) for genetic defects statistics (including cystic fibrosis). Chargaff (1973) discusses the revulsion from science. I. Chalmers (1976) described the Oxford criticism; in this regard, see also Chard (1977). The news report in the Bangladesh Times was written by Zagrulla·Chowdry. See Annotation (1974) for recommendations of the West African workshop. Mumford (1946) discussed a program for survival. See Editorial (1977) for comments about malpractice trials. See Lowenfeld (1975) for an account of the independence movement among the blind. See Commoner (1973) for comments on the social responsibility of science. See Hunter (1978) for the North Carolina study of social chaos in families of ex-premature infants. See Lehrer (1965) for his song, *That Was the Year That Was*. See Brody (1973) for a discussion of the distinction between technical problems and value problems. Freidson's book (1972) is an excellent sociologic analysis of the profession of medicine. See WHO report (1976) for the role of physicians in ethical problems related to birth defects. Lawless (1974) commented on "Medical Practice." The "Values Underlying . . ." conference was reported by Steinfels (1978). See Firth (1970) for the effects of evangelism in Tikopia. Webster (1976) described the Puritan outlook on science and medicine. See Mumford (1970) for brilliant comments on the growth of technology. See Watch Tower (undated) and Frankel (1977) for the attitudes of Jehovah's Witnesses concerning blood transfusion. See Brody (1973) as in the above-cited quote. G.B. Shaw's maxim appears in the epilogue of *Man and Superman*. See von Fritz (1952) for a discussion of relative and absolute values. See Kluckhohn (1951) for the definition and comments about morals in an excellent essay which gives an anthropologist's analysis of the concept of values. See Beecher (1966) for the classification of clinical studies. The Anti-Vivisection Society's brochure was sent to me some time in the 1960s. See Schulman (1967) for the presidential address to the Society for Pediatric Research. See Gregory (1971) for the continuous positive airway pressure report, and Surgeon-General (1966) for the Public Health Service memorandum concerning signed informed consent. The "While controlled trials . . ." quote is from Stern (1975). See Bernard (1865) for the "Many physicians attack . . ." quote.

Chapter 13   The Experimental Method in
Clinical Studies of Children

The material in this chapter will appear, in different form, in my book on human experimentation insthe Scientific American Illustrated Library series. See Smithells (1975) for the "I need permission . . ." quote. See Singer (1976) for comments about the orientation of bioethecists. Cahn (1972) described the "Pompey Syndrome"; the passage is reproduced with permission of the original publisher, copyright The Johns Hopkins University Press 1964. See Greenwood (1942-43) and Graunt (1662) for the origins of medical statistics. Bronowski (1977) discussed the development of the experimental method. Claude Bernard's quotes are from his book (1865). See Freidson (1972) for his comments. See Bronowski (1959) for the quote concerning the statistical method. In this regard, no less a personage than Albert Einstein resisted the use of the statistical approach to explore natural (subatomic) events, with his famous remark, "God does not play dice with the world." The quote attributed to Galen is found in Strauss (1968). The South Pacific story is apocryphal. See Venn (1866) for the most lucid discussion of the logic of chance extant (!); the description of the behavior of observations in a *series* is taken from his classic book. Gauss' Law expresses the number of errors (variations) of each size that are expected to occur as the result of chance in many measurable characteristics appearing in nature and in the man-made world. For example, in target shooting, the hits group themselves in a pattern: close to the bullseye they are densely packed, farther from it there are fewer and fewer hits, until there are none at all. The frequency distribution, when plotted out according to the distances that separate the hits from the bullseye, has the physical appearance of the familiar bell-shaped figure: the Gaussian normal curve. The mathematical equation of this curve (which includes the two parameters of the equation: the central value of the distribution expressed as the arithmetic mean and the dispersion of values around the mean expressed as the standard deviation) provides the basis for the arithmetic operations used in making statistical inferences about the variations with a *similar* distribution which occur in a series of observations. These variations occur in the field of measurements (e.g., stature, concentration of substances in the blood, cognitive tests). They also appear as vairations in the proportions of dichotomous characteristics (qualities which divide the "population" into two mutually exclusive groups) in a series seen in medical problems (e.g., "alive" or "dead", "RLF" or "no-RLF" . . .) and in gambling problems (e.g., "heads" or "tails" in coin-tossing). See Levinson (1939) for a most readable account of gambling and the laws of chance. The probability that two successive events both take place is equal to the probability of the first event multiplied by the second (the latter being computed on the assumption that the first event has already taken place). The probability of "heads" on a single toss of a coin is ½ and the chance of throwing two successive "heads" in two tosses is $(\frac{1}{2})^2 = \frac{1}{4}$. The general rule for calculating the chance of throwing any number of n successive "heads" in n tosses is $(\frac{1}{2})^n$. And the chance of throwing a number of "heads" in a succession during a long series of tosses is calculated from the formula $(\frac{1}{2})^{n+2}$ For two successive "heads" the computation is $(\frac{1}{2})^{2+2}$ $=0.0625$; thus, in a set of 100 tosses of the coin about 6 runs of two-heads-in-a-row are expected. See Fisher (1925 and 1926) for a description of his field-experiment designs. See Hill (1937 and 1953) for his early writings; a description of the classic streptomycin trial is reprinted in Hill (1962). The MRC streptomycin trial is usually cited as the first of its kind because it kindled considerable interest and led directly to further studies on the same model. It is unfortunate that previous well-planned controlled clinical trials (see Amberson 1931 and Patulin Clinical Trials Committee 1944) did not stimulate widespread interest in the power of this study format. I believe this was related to the fact that the early trials were negative: they failed to demonstrate the effectiveness of proposed treatments (sodium-gold-thiosulphate treatment of tuberculosis in 1931, and a metabolic product of *Penicillin patulin,* called "patulin," for the treatment of the common cold in 1944). See Mainland (1952), Feinstein (1977) and Sackett (1975) for discussions of methodologic issues in clinical experimentation. See Mainland (1960) for examples of misuse of statistical arithmetic. See Bronowski (1977) for the comment about Darwin. See Cochrane (1972) for the coronary-care-units story. Byar (1976) discussed the problems of adaptive designs. See T.C. Chalmers (1975) for comments about randomization. The task force findings on risks for human subjects was reported by Cardon (1976). The comments of the Boston group appeared in a letter to the editor (Boston Interhospital 1975). See Fried (1974) for a discussion of legal issues. See Kabat (1975) for his questions. See Selvin (1966) for "data-dredging." See Kinsey (1977) for the results of the blood oxygen study. See Eisenberg (1977) concerning the social need to foster excellence in medical research. See Popper (1962) for his comment.

Chapter 14 The Future for Studies Involving American Children

See Price (1961 and 1963) for his analysis of the growth of science; Fig. 14-1A is redrawn from his book (1961) and Fig. 14-1B is redrawn from Durack (1978). Price points out that logistic curves of growth have become well known in numerous analyses of time series, especially those concerning the growth of science and technology. See Mahler (1977) for comments on health care development. See Tuskegee (undated) for conclusions after investigating policies to protect research subjects. See Eisenberg (1977) for his comment. Meier (1972) summarized the experience of the 1954 polio vaccine trials. Comroe (1976) reported the review of the key research efforts leading to the ten most important advances. The "Lyndon Johnson doctrine" phrase is Eisenberg's (1977). See Bronowski (1977) for a dicussion of society's involvement with science, and Medawar (1969) for the history of development of the scientific method. Juhl (1977) reported the "epidemiology" of the randomized clinical trial (in gastroenterology), and Tannenbaum (1977) reported the survey in institutions conducting research in children. See Walster (1970) for the editorial policy proposal. See Barber (1973) for discussion of clinical research among the poor. See Jonas (1970) for a discussion of recruitment of subjects for experimentation. In connection with experimentation in the children of physicians, see Altman (1972). Claude Bernard's maxim appears in his book (1865). See National Commission (1977) for recommendations concerning research involving children, and American Academy (1977) for guidelines developed by the American Academy of Pediatrics. Jonas (1970) has given considerable thought to the agonizing question of whom should be called upon to participate in clinical studies. See Bostock (1962) for the "exterior gestation" thesis, and Klaus (1976) for evidence concerning the dyadic relationship between mother and infant. Ramsay (1970), Bartholome (1977) and Hauerwas (1977) have written about the rights of the fetus and the newborn. See Eisenberg (1977) for his comments about informed consent. Guttentag (1953) discussed the problem of experimentation on human beings years before the present-day crisis. We began to implement his suggestions about 9 months before the National Institutes (1953) guidelines were circulated, see Silverman (1966). T.C. Chalmers (1974) reviewed the DES incident and other examples of the alienation of practicing physicians from research results. Two marketing surveys provided the estimates of DES usage in the 1960-70 period, see Heinonen (1973). Mahler (1977) recommended community trials. Popper's book, *The Logic of Scientific Discovery*, was published in German in 1934; it was not translated into English for 25 years (see Popper 1959 and 1962). See Bronowski (1977) for a critique of Popper's test-by-refutation proposal and Perkinson (1978) for an excellent summary of the Popperian approach. In connection with failures to confirm an hypothesis, the use of the term "no significant difference" introduces confusion, unless otherwise qualified. A. Bradford Hill once advised:

. . . it is better (particularly in a matter of importance) to take "statistically not significant" as the "non-proven" of Scot's Law rather than as the "not-guilty" of English Law.

The phrase "no significant difference" may denote (1) a difference which is no greater than would be expected reasonably often in repeated sets of observations of a given size solely as the result of random variation (for example, the true difference in survival between two methods of care is zero), or (2) a difference which is not important to the community [for example, the true difference in survival is not zero, but it is so small that (a), it does not justify investment of the available resources of the community, or (b), for practical purposes the two methods of care may be considered equal alternatives]. If the number of observations is few the true difference may be quite large and the decision "no significant difference" is reached because of an inappropriately small sample size. In clinical trials, estimates of sample size "needed" are determined on the basis of more or less arbitrary answers to questions posed *before the trial begins:* (1) What shall be considered an important difference, for example, in survival? (2) What risk of errors shall be assumed (a) to declare a "difference" when the true increase in survival is zero, and (b) to declare "no significant difference" when the true difference is as great or greater than the important amount? Concerning a critical test of oxygen curtailment in the first two days of life, it is interesting to turn back to an editorial written in November 1954, two months after the announcement of the results of the Cooperative Study (see Gordon 1954b). After reviewing the evidence concerning oxygen treatment of premature infants up to that time, Doctor Gordon noted that ". . . until carefully controlled studies of oxygen therapy . . . are available, empiric evidence . . . must be used to guide physicians in the treatment of these babies during the first 48 hours of life." The "carefully controlled studies" were never carried out. Claude Bernard's quote appears in his book (1865).

Appendices

See Zacharias (1952) for the information in Appendix A. See Kinsey (1956a) for details in Appendices B and C. See Sackett (1975) for the methodologic standards in Appendix D.

BIBLIOGRAPHY

Akeson N
1976   What is the current incidence of RLF? Pediatrics 58:627

Agerty HA and Seitchik JN
1952   Experimental use of methyl testosterone and testosterone in premature infants. Pediatrics 10:28–32

Alexander HE
1957   in Day RL and Silverman WA: Premature and newborn infants. Report of a seminar. Pediatrics 20:143–154

Allen FH and Diamond LK
1958   Erythroblastosis Fetalis. Little Brown, Boston

Altman LK
1972   Auto-experimentation. An unappreciated tradition in medical science. New Engl J Med 286:346–352

Amberson JB et al.
1931   A clinical trial of sanocrysin in pulmonary tuberculosis. Am Rev Tuberculosis 24:401–435

American Academy of Pediatrics, Committee on Drugs
1977   Guidelines for the ethical conduct of studies to evaluate drugs in pediatric populations. Pediatrics 60:91–101

Andrews BF et al.
1965   Effects of hypertonic magnesium-sulfate enemas on newborn and young lambs. Lancet 2:64–65

Annotation
1974   Management in Africa. Lancet 2:1301–1302

Annotation
1975   Postscript to thalidomide. Lancet 1:560

Aranda JV et al.
1975   Blood transfusion: Possible potentiating risk factor in retrolental fibroplasia. Pediat Res 9:362

Ashton N, Ward B and Serpell G
1953   Role of oxygen in the genesis of retrolental fibroplasia. A preliminary report. Brit J Ophth 37:513–520

1954   Effect of oxygen on developing retinal vessels with particular
            reference to the problem of retrolental fibroplasia. Brit J
            Ophth 38:397–432

Ashton N
1964   Personal communication cited in Tizard J P M: Indications for
            oxygen therapy in the newborn. Pediatrics 34:771–786
1966   Oxygen and growth and development of retinal vessels. Am J
            Ophth 62:412–435

Ashton N and Henkind P
1965   Experimental occlusion of retinal arterioles: Using graded
            glass ballotini. Brit J Ophth 49:225–234

Ashton N
1970   Retinal angiogenesis in the human embryo. Brit Med Bull
            26:103–106

Avery ME and Oppenheimer EH
1960   Recent increase in mortality from hyaline membrane disease. J
            Pediatrics 57:553–559

Bakwin H
1923   Oxygen therapy in premature infants with anoxemia. Am J Dis
            Child 25:157–162

Balentine JD and Gutsche BB
1966   Central nervous system lesions in rats exposed to oxygen at
            high pressure. Am J Pathology 48:107–127

Ballantyne JW
1902   The problem of the premature infant. Lancet 1:1196–1200

Barber B et al.
1973   Research on Human Subjects. Problems of Social Control in
            Medical Experimentation. Russell Sage Foundation, New York

Bartholome WG
1977   Proxy consent in the medical context: the infant as a person, in
            Appendix to Report and Recommendations on Research In-
            volving Children of the National Commission for the Protec-
            tion of Human Subjects . . . etc. DHEW Publication No. (OS)
            77-0005

Baum JD
1971a   Retinal artery tortuosity in ex-premature infants. 18-year fol-

low-up on eyes of premature infants. Arch Dis Child 46: 247–252

1971b   Retinal photography in premature infants: *forme fruste* retrolental fibroplasia. Roy Soc Med (London) 64:777–779

1977   The continuum of caretaking casualty. Dev Med Child Neurol 19:543–544

Bedrossian RH et al.

1954   Retinopathy of prematurity (retrolental fibroplasia) and oxygen. Am J Ophth 37:78–86

Beecher, HK

1966   Ethics and clinical research. New Engl J Med 274:1354–1360

Belenky DA et al.

1978   Unconvinced by CDP evidence (letter). Pediatrics 61:500–501

Bernard C

1865   An Introduction to the Study of Experimental Medicine (transl. by HC Greene). Henry Schuman, Inc., New York

Bloxom A

1950   Resuscitation of the newborn infant. Use of the positive pressure oxygen-air lock. J Pediatrics 37:311–319

Bolton DPG and Cross KW

1974   Further observations on cost of preventing retrolental fibroplasia. Lancet 1:445–448

Bostock J

1962   Evolutional approach to infant care. Lancet 1:1033–1035

Boston Interhospital Virus Study Group

1975   Delaying double-blind drug evaluation in usually fatal diseases. (Letter) New Engl J Med 293:509

Briggs JN

1955   A clinical trial of Alevaire in pulmonary distress of the newborn infant. J Pediatrics 46:621–625

Brody H

1973   The systems view of man: Implications for medicine, science and ethics. Perspect Biol Med 17:71–92

Broman S, Nichols PL and Kennedy WA

1975   Preschool I.Q.—Prenatal and Early Developmental Correlates. Erlbaum Assoc., Hillsdale, New Jersey

Bronowski J
  1959   The Common Sense of Science. Random House, New York
  1977   A Sense of the Future, MIT Press, Cambridge, MA

Budin P
  1900   Le Nourisson, Octave Doin, Paris (English transl by WJ
           Maloney: The Nursling. The Caxton Publ. Co., London, 1907)

Burns LE et al.
  1959   Fatal circulatory collapse in premature infants receiving chlor-
           amphenicol. New Engl J Med 261:1318– 1321

Byar DP et al.
  1976   Randomized clinical trials. Perspectives on some recent ideas.
           New Engl J Med 295:74– 80

Cahn E
  1972   Drug experiments and the public conscience, quoted in Katz
           J.: Experimentation with Human Beings. Russell Sage Foun-
           dation, New York

Campbell K
  1951   Intensive oxygen therapy as a possible cause of retrolental
           fibroplasia: A clinical approach. Med J Australia 2:48– 50

Campbell FW
  1951   The influence of a low atmospheric pressure on the develop-
           ment of the retinal vessels in the rat. Tr Ophth Soc U Kingdom
           71:287– 300

Cardon PV et al.
  1976   Injuries to research subjects: a survey of investigators. New
           Engl J Med 295:650– 654

Chalmers I
  1976   British debate on obstetric practice. Pediatrics 58:308– 312

Chalmers TC
  1974   The impact of controlled trials on the practice of medicine. Mt
           Sinai J Med 41:753– 758
  1975   Randomization: Perils and problems (Letter). New Engl J Med
           292:1036– 1037

Chapple CC
  1938   An incubator for infants. Am J Obstet Gynecol 35:1062– 1065

Chard T and Richards M (eds.)
  1977   Benefits and Hazards of the New Obstetrics. Spastics Int.
          Med. Publ., London

Chargaff E
  1973   Bitter fruits from the tree of knowledge: Remarks on the cur-
          rent revulsion from science. Perspect Biol Med 16:486–502
  1976   Triviality in science: A brief meditation on fashions. Persp
          Biol Med 19:324–333

Chase JB
  1972   Retrolental Fibroplasia and Autistic Symptomatology. Ameri-
          can Foundation For Blind, New York

Chu J et al.
  1967   Neonatal pulmonary ischemia. Part I. Clinical and physiolog-
          ical studies. Pediatrics 40:709–782

Clark LC
  1956   The control and monitoring of blood and tissue oxygen. Trans
          Amer Soc Int Org 2:41–48

Clifford SH
  1950   Prevention and control of infection in nurseries for premature
          infants. Am J Dis Child 79:377–383

Cochrane AL
  1972   Effectiveness and Efficiency. Random Reflections on Health
          Services. Nuffield Provincial Hospitals Trust, London

Cogan DG
  1963   Development and senescence of human retinal vasculature.
          Trans Ophth Soc U Kingdom 83:465–489

Coleman J et al.
  1957   The diffusion of an innovation among physicians. Sociometry
          20:253–270

Collins ET and Mayou MS
  1925   Pathology and Bacteriology of the Eye, 2nd Ed. Blakiston's
          Sons, Philadelphia

Commentary
  1897   The use of incubators for infants. Lancet 1:1490

Commoner B
  1973   The responsibility of science. New York Times, August 12,
          1973, p 15

Comroe JH and Dripps RD
    1976   Scientific basis for the support of biomedical science. Science
             192:105–111

Cross KW
    1973   Cost of preventing retrolental fibroplasia? Lancet 2:954–956

Crosse VM
    1951   The problem of retrolental fibroplasia in the city of Birming-
             ham. Tr Ophth Soc U Kingdom 71:609–612

Davies DP
    1978   The first feed of low birthweight infants: Changing attitudes in
             the twentieth century. Arch Dis Child 53:187–192

Davies PA
    1976   Outlook for the low birthweight baby—then and now. Arch
             Dis Child 51:817–819

Day RL et al.
    1979   Interpretation of statistical nonsignificance and retrolental fib-
             roplasia. Pediatrics 63:342–343

Denucé J
    1857   Note sur quelques faits de practique Chirurgicale. J Med Bor-
             deaux 2:723

Donald I
    1954   Augmented respiration: An emergency positive-pressure pa-
             tient-cycled respirator. Lancet 1:895–899

Dormandy TL
    1978   Free-radical oxidation and antioxidants. Lancet 1:647–650

Drillien CM
    1961   The incidence of mental and physical handicaps in school-age
             children of very low birthweight. Pediatrics 27:452–464
    1967   The long-term prospects for babies of low birth weight. Hospi-
             tal Medicine (London) 1:937–944

Dunham E
    1957   Evolution of premature infant care. Ann Paediat Fenn 3:170–
             184

Durack DT
    1978   The weight of medical knowledge. New Engl J Med 298:
             773–775

Editorial
   1974   Retrolental fibroplasia (RLF) unrelated to oxygen therapy.
               Brit J Ophth 58:487–489
   1977   Blind justice. Pediatrics 59:781–782

Eisenberg L
   1977   The social imperatives of medical research. Science 198:1105–
               1110

Elonen AS and Zwarensteyn SB
   1964   Appraisal of developmental lag in certain blind children. J
               Pediatrics 65:599–610

Erbe RW
   1977   Genetic disorders, in Wechsler H et al: Horizons of Health.
               Harvard University Press, Cambridge, MA

Evans PJ
   1951   Retrolental fibroplasia. Tr Ophth Soc U Kingdom 71:613–616

Exline Jr. AL and Harrington MR
   1951   Retrolental fibroplasia; clinical statistics from the premature
               center of Charity Hospital of Louisiana at New Orleans. J
               Pediatrics 38:1–7

Feeney L and Berman ER
   1976   Oxygen toxicity: Membrane damage by free radicals. Invest
               Ophthalmology 15:789–792

Feinstein AR
   1977   Clinical Biostatistics. Mosby, St Louis, MO

Finberg L
   1967   Dangers to infants caused by changes in osmolal concentra-
               tion. Pediatrics 40:1031–1034

Firth R
   1970   Rank and Religion in Tikopia. Beacon Press, Boston, MA

Fisher RA
   1925   Statistical Methods for Research Workers. Oliver and Boyd,
               Edinburgh
   1926   The arrangement of field experiments. J Ministry Agric 33:
               503–506
   1949   The Design of Experiments, 5th Ed. Oliver and Boyd, Edin-
               burgh

Flynn JT et al.
1977   Retrolental fibroplasia. I. Clinical observations. Arch Ophth
          95:217–223

Fraiberg S
1977   Insights From the Blind. Basic Books, New York

Frankel LS et al.
1977   Childhood cancer and the Jehovah's Witness faith. Pediatrics
          60:916–921

Freidson E
1972   Profession of Medicine. Dodd, Mead & Co., New York

Fried C
1974   Medical Experimentation: Personal Integrity and Social Poli-
          cy. American Elsevier, New York

Fürst L
1887   Ueber Warmervorrichthungen für zu frühgeborne oder lebens-
          schwache. Kinder Dtsch Med Wschr 13:772–775

Gaull GE et al.
1977   Milk protein quantity and quality in low-birth-weight infants.
          III. Effects on sulfur amino acids in plasma and urine. J Pedi-
          atrics 90:348–355

Gleiss J
1955   Zum Frühgeborenenproblem der Gegenwart: IX. Mitteilung.
          Über fütterungs und umweltbedingte Atemstörungen bei Früh-
          geborenen. Ztschr Kinderh 76:261–268

Gordon HH and McNamara H
1941   Fat excretion of premature infants. I. Effects on fecal fat of
          decreasing fat intake. Am J Dis Child 62:328–345

Gordon HH, Lubchenco L and Hix I
1954a   Observations on the etiology of retrolental fibroplasia. Bull
          Johns Hopkins Hosp 94:34–44

Gordon HH
1954b   Oxygen administration and retrolental fibroplasia. Editorial
          Comment. Pediatrics 14:543–546
1957   Oxygen therapy and survival rate in prematures (Letter). Pedi-
          atrics 19:967

Graunt J
1662   Natural and Political Observations Made Upon the Bills of

Mortality. Edited by Walter Willcox. Johns Hopkins University Press, Baltimore, 1939

Greenwood M
1942-43 Medical statistics from Graunt to Farr. Biometrika 32:101–127, 32:203–225 and 33:1–24

Gregory GA et al.
1971   Treatment of the idiopathic respiratory-distress syndrome with continuous positive airway pressure. New Engl J Med 284: 1333–1340

Grove RD and Hetzell AM
1968   Vital Statistics Rates in the United States 1940–1960. PHS Publication No. 1677

Grumbach MM et al.
1959   On the fetal masculinizing action of certain oral progestins. J Clin Endocrinol 19:1369–1380

Guttentag OE
1953   The problem of experimentation on human beings. II. The physician's point of view. Science 117:207–210

Guy LP et al.
1956   The possibility of total elimination of retrolental fibroplasia by oxygen restriction. Pediatrics 17:247–249

Gyllensten LJ and Hellström BE
1952   Retrolental fibroplasia—animal experiments. Acta Paediat 41: 577–582
1956   IV. The effects of gradual and of rapid transfer from concentrated oxygen to normal air on the oxygen induced changes in the eyes of young mice. Am J Ophth 41:619–627

Gyllensten LJ
1959   Influence of oxygen exposure on the postnatal vascularization of the cerebral cortex in mice. Acta Morph Neerl Scand 2: 289–310

Harris M
1977   Cannibals and Kings. Random House, New York

Hatfield EM
1972   Blindness in infants and young children. Sightsav Rev 42: 69–89

    1975   Why are they blind? Sightsav Rev 45:3–22

Hauerwas S
    1977   Rights, duties, and experimentation in children, in Appendix
                to Report and Recommendations on Research Involving Chil-
                dren of the National Commission for the Protection of Human
                Subjects . . . etc. DHEW Publication No. (OS) 77-0005

Heinonen OP
    1973   Diethylstilbestrol in pregnancy. Frequency of exposure and
                usage patterns. Cancer 31:573–577

Hellman L
    1976   Scoundrel Time. Little Brown and Co., Boston

Hepner Jr. WR
    1952   Retrolental fibroplasia in premature infants and in kittens (Ab-
                stract). Am J Dis Child 84:748

Hess JH
    1922   Premature and Congenitally Diseased Infants. Lea & Febiger,
                Philadelphia

Hess JH et al.
    1934a   The Physical and Mental Growth of Prematurely Born Chil-
                dren. University of Chicago Press, Chicago

Hess JH
    1934b   Oxygen unit for premature and very young infants. Am J Dis
                Child 47:916–917

Hill AB
    1937   Principles of Medical Statistics. Oxford University Press,
                New York
    1953   The Philosophy of the Clinical Trial. N.I.H. Annual Lectures.
                PHS Publications No. 388, U.S. Govt. Printing Office, Wash-
                ington
    1962   Statistical Methods in Clinical and Preventive Medicine. Ox-
                ford University Press, New York

Hinds MW
    1974   Fewer doctors and infant survival (Letter). New Engl J Med
                291:741

Hobel CJ et al.
    1972   An early versus late treatment of neonatal acidosis in low-
                birth-weight infants: Relation to respiratory distress syndrome.
                J Pediatrics 81:1178–1187

Houlton ACL
  1951   A study of cases of retrolental fibroplasia seen in Oxford. Tr
          Ophth Soc U Kingdom 71:583–590

Huch A, Huch R and Lucey JF (eds)
  1979   Continuous Transcutaneous Blood Gas Monitoring. Alan R.
          Liss, Inc., New York

Huch R, Huch A and Lübbers DW
  1973   Transcutaneous measurement of blood PO_2 ($TcPO_2$). Method
          and application in perinatal medicine. J Perinat Med 1:183–191

Hunter RS et al.
  1978   Antecedents of child abuse in premature infants: A prospective
          study in a newborn intensive care unit. Pediatrics 61:629–635

Hurlin RC
  1962   Estimated prevalence of blindness in the United States and in
          individual states, 1960. Sightsav Rev 32:4–12

Ingalls TH
  1948   Congenital encephalo-ophthalmic dysplasia. Pediatrics 1:
          315–325

Ingalls TH et al.
  1952   Congenital malformations of the eye induced in mice by ma-
          ternal anoxia. With particular reference to the problem of ret-
          rolental fibroplasia in man. Am J Ophth 35:311–329

Insight Team of The Sunday Times of London
  1979   Suffer the Children: The Story of Thalidomide. Viking Press,
          New York

James LS and Lanman JT
  1976   History of oxygen therapy and retrolental fibroplasia. Pediat-
          rics 57(Suppl):591–642

Johnson L et al.
  1974   The premature infant, vitamin E deficiency and retrolental
          fibroplasia. Am J Clin Nutr 27:1158–1173

Jonas H
  1970   Philosophical reflections on human experimentation, in Freund

PA; Experimentation with Human Subjects. Braziller, New York

Jonsen A et al.
  1975   Critical issues in newborn intensive care. Pediatrics 55:756–768

Jordan TE
  1970   Early developmental adversity program (EDAP) #17: A neonatal cohort at forty-two months. Central Midwest Regional Educational Laboratory (CMREL), St Louis

Juhl E et al.
  1977   The epidemiology of the gastrointestinal randomized clinical trial. New Engl J Med 296:20–22

Kabat EA
  1975   Ethics and the wrong answer (Editorial). Science 189:505

Katz J
  1972   Experimentation with Human Beings. Russell Sage Foundation, New York

Kingham JD
  1977   Acute retrolental fibroplasia. Arch Ophth 95:39–47

Kinsey VE and Zacharias L
  1949   Retrolental fibroplasia: Incidence in different localities in recent years and a correlation of the incidence with treatment given the infants. JAMA 139:572–578

Kinsey VE and Chisholm Jr. JF
  1951   Retrolental fibroplasia: Evaluation of several changes in dietary supplements of premature infants with respect to the incidence of the disease. Am J Ophth 34:1259–1268

Kinsey VE
  1955   Etiology of retrolental fibroplasia and preliminary report of the Cooperative Study of Retrolental Fibroplasia. Tr Am Acad Ophth Otol 59:15–24
  1956a   Retrolental fibroplasia. Cooperative study of retrolental fibroplasia and the use of oxygen. AMA Arch Ophth 56:481–543
  1956b   Caution in oxygen therapy to prevent retrolental fibroplasia (Letter). Pediatrics 18:511

Kinsey VE et al.
1977   PaO₂ levels and retrolental fibroplasia. A report of the cooper-
         ative study. Pediatrics 60:655–667

Klaus MH and Kennell JH
1976   Maternal–infant Bonding. CV Mosby, St Louis

Kluckhohn C et al.
1951   Values and value-orientations in the theory of action. An ex-
         ploration in definition and classification. In Parsons T and
         Schills EA: Toward a General Theory of Action. Harvard Uni-
         versity Press, Cambridge, MA

Krause AC
1946   Congenital encephalo-ophthalmic dysplasia. Arch Ophth 36:
         387–444

Kushner BJ et al.
1977   Retrolental fibroplasia. II. Pathologic correlation. Arch Ophth
         95:29–38

Lanman JT et al.
1954   Retrolental fibroplasia and oxygen therapy. JAMA 155:223–
         226

Lanman JT
1955   The control of oxygen therapy for premature infants. Health
         News 32:14–16

Lawless J and Lawless M
1974   Protein requirement (Letter). Lancet 2:947–948

Lee KL et al.
1976   Determinants of the neonatal mortality. Am J Dis Child 130:
         842–845

Lehrer T
1965   Wernher von Braun, in Reprise Record 6179: *That Was the
         Year That Was*

Lelong M et al.
1952   Sur la retinopathic des prematures (fibroplasie retrolentale).
         Arch Franc Pediat 9:897–915

Levinson HC
1939   The Science of Chance. Rinehart, New York

Lipton EL et al.
  1965   Swaddling, child-care practice: Historical, cultural and exper-
            imental observations. Pediatrics 35 (Suppl):521–567

Locke JC and Reese AB
  1952   Retrolental fibroplasia. The negative role of light, mydriatics,
            and the ophthalmoscope examination in its etiology. AMA
            Arch Ophth 48:44–47

Lowenfeld B
  1947   The Pre-School Child. American Foundation for the Blind,
            New York
  1959   Observations on incidence and effects of retrolental fibroplasia.
            New Outlook Blind 53:15–19
  1975   The Changing Status of the Blind. Chas C. Thomas, Spring-
            field, IL

MacMahon B and Berlin JE
  1977   Health of the United States population, in Wechsler H et al:
            Horizons of Health. Harvard University Press, Cambridge,
            MA

McCormick AQ
  1977   Retinopathy of prematurity. Current Probl Pediat 7:3–28

McDonald AD
  1962   Neurological and ophthalmic disorders in children of very low
            birth weight. Brit Med J 1:895–900

McKeown T
  1976   The Modern Rise of Population. Academic Press, New York

Mahler H
  1977   Problems of medical affluence. WHO Chronicle 31:8–13

Mainland D
  1952   Elementary Medical Statistics. WB Saunders, Philadelphia
  1960   The use and misuse of statistics in medical publications (Com-
            mentary). Clin Pharmacol Therapy 1:411–422

Mann I
  1928   Development of the Human Eye. Oxford University Press,
            Cambridge

Medawar PB
  1969   Induction and Intuition in Scientific Thought. American Phil-
            osophical Society, Philadelphia

Meier P
   1972   The biggest public health experiment ever, in Tanur JM (ed):
             Statistics: A Guide to the Unknown. Holden-Day, Inc., San
             Francisco

Meissner FL
   1838   Die kinderkrankheiten nach neusten Ansichten und Erfahrun-
             gen zum Unterricht fur practische Aertze. List, Leipzig

Menkes JH, Chernick V and Ringel B
   1966   Effect of elevated blood tyrosine on subsequent intellectual
             development of premature infants. J Pediatrics 69:583–588

Meyer TC and Angus J
   1956   The effect of large doses of "synkavit" in the newborn. Arch
             Dis Child 31:212–215

Michaelson IC
   1948   Vascular morphogeneis in the retina of the cat. J Anat 82:
             167–174
   1954   Retinal Circulation in Man and Animals. Chas C. Thomas,
             Springfield, IL

Miller Jr. JA
   1957   Influence of temperature upon resistance to asphyxia, in John-
             son FH: Influence of Temperature on Biological Systems.
             Williams and Wilkins, Baltimore

Millcn RS et al.
   1955   Prevention of neonatal asphyxia with the use of a rocking
             resuscitator. Am J Obstet Gynecol 70:1087–1091

Moore TD (ed)
   1976   Iatrogenic Problems in Neonatal Intensive Care. Report of the
             Sixty-Ninth Conference on Pediatric Research. Ross Labora-
             tories, Columbus, Ohio

Morris NM et al.
   1975   Shifting age-parity distribution of births and the decrease in
             infant mortality. Am J Public Health 65:359–362

Mumford L
   1946   Program for survival, in Values for Survival. Harcourt, Brace
             and Co., New York
   1970   The Myth of the Machine. The Pentagon of Power. Harcourt,
             Brace Jovanovich, New York

Murphy RJ
  1951   North Carolina premature infant program. North Carolina Med J
            12:12–18

Mushin AS
  1974   Retinopathy of prematurity—a disease of increasing incidence.
            Tr Ophth Soc U Kingdom 94:251–253

Naftulin DH et al.
  1973   The Doctor Fox lecture: A paradigm of educational seduction.
            J Med Educ 48:630–635

National Commission for the Protection of Human Subjects of Biomedical
and Behavioral Research
  1977   Report and Recommendations: Research Involving Children.
            DHEW No. (OS) 77-0004, Washington

National Center for Health Statistics
  1977   Vital Statistics of the United States 1973. Vol. 1 DHEW No.
            HRA 77-113

National Institutes of Health
  1953   Informed understanding (Memorandum). November 17, 1953

Neligan G et al.
  1974   The Formative Years. Oxford University Press, London

Outerbridge EW et al.
  1973   Magnesium sulfate enema in a newborn. Fatal systemic mag-
            nesium absorption. JAMA 224:1392–1393

Owens WC and Owens EU
  1948   Retrolental fibroplasia in premature infants. Tr Am Acad Ophth
            Otol 53:18–41
  1949a   Retrolental fibroplasia in premature infants. Am J Ophth 32:
            1–21
  1949b   Retrolental fibroplasia in premature infants: II. Studies on the
            prophylaxis of the disease; The use of alpha tocopheryl [sic]
            acetate. Am J Ophth 32:1631–1637

Owens WC
  1953   Spontaneous regression in retrolental fibroplasia. Tr Am Ophth
            Soc 51:555–579

Pakter J and Jacobziner H
    1954   A five-year review of the premature infant program in New York City. NY State J Med 54:3207–3215

Pakter J and Nelson F
    1974   Factors in the unprecedented decline in infant mortality in New York City. Bull NY Acad Med 50:839–867

Patulin Clinical Trials Committee
    1944   Clinical trial of patulin in the common cold. Lancet 2:373–375

Patz A et al.
    1952   Studies on the effect of high oxygen administration in retrolental fibroplasia. I. Nursery observations. Am J Ophth 35:1248–1253

Patz A et al.
    1953   Oxygen studies in retrolental fibroplasia. II. The production of the microscopic changes of retrolental fibroplasia in experimental animals. Am J Ophth 36:1511–1522

Patz A
    1955   Experimental studies, in Symposium on retrolental fibroplasia. Tr Am Acad Ophth 59:25–34
    1957a   The role of oxygen in retrolental fibroplasia. Pediatrics 19:504–524

Patz A and Eastham AB
    1957b   Oxygen studies in retrolental fibroplasia. V. The effect of rapid vs. gradual withdrawal from oxygen on the mouse eye. AMA Arch Ophth 57:724–729

Peller S
    1948   Mortality, past and future. Pop Studies 1:405–456

Perkinson H
    1978   Popper's fallibilism. Et Cetera 35:3–19

Phelps DL and Rosenbaum AL
    1977   The role of tocopherol in oxygen-induced retinopathy: Kitten model. Pediatrics 59(Suppl):998–1005

Pomerance JJ et al.
    1978   Cost of living for infants weighing 1000 grams or less at birth. Pediatrics 61:908–910

Popper KR
    1959   The Logic of Scientific Study. Basic Books, New York

1962   Conjectures and Refutations: The Growth of Scientific Know-
        ledge. Basic Books, New York

Powell H et al.
1973   Hexachlorophene myelinopathy in premature infants. J Pediat-
        rics 82:976–981

Price DJ de S
1961   Science Since Babylon. Yale University Press, New Haven
1963   Little Science, Big Science. Columbia University Press, New
        York

Ramsey P
1970   The Patient as a Person. Yale University Press, New Haven

Ravenel SF
1953   New techniques of humidification in pediatrics. JAMA 151:
        707–711

Reese AB
1949   Persistence and hyperplasia of primary vitreous; retrolental
        fibroplasia—two entities. Arch Ophth 41:527–549

Reese AB and Blodi FC
1951   Retrolental fibroplasia. Am J Ophth 34:1–24

Reichelderfer TE and Nitowsky HM
1956   A controlled study of the use of the Bloxom air lock. Pediatrics
        18:918–927

Roberton NRC et al.
1968   Oxygen therapy in the newborn. Lancet 1:1323–1329

Ryan H
1952   Retrolental fibroplasia, a clinicopathologic study. Am J Ophth
        35:329–342

Sackett DL
1975   Design, measurement and analysis in clinical trials, in Hirsch
        J: Platelets, Drugs, and Thrombosis. Karger, Basle, Switzerland

Sameroff AJ and Chandler MJ
1975   Reproductive risk and the continuum of caretaking casualty,
        in Horowitz FD (ed): Review of Child Development Research.
        University of Chicago Press, Chicago

Sandars TC
  1876   The Institutes of Justinian. Callaghan, Chicago

Schulman I
  1967   Clinical investigation in children. Pediat Res 1:196–199

Selvin HC and Stuart A
  1966   Data-dredging procedures in survey analysis. Am Statistician
            20:20–23

Shapiro S et al.
  1968   Infant, Perinatal, Maternal, and Childhood Mortality in the
            United States. Harvard University Press, Cambridge, MA

Silverman WA et al.
  1955   Controlled clinical trial of effects of Alevaire mist on prema-
            ture infants. JAMA 157:1093–1096
  1956a   A controlled clinical trial of effects of water mist on obstruc-
            tive respiratory signs, death rate and necropsy findings among
            premature infants. Pediatrics 17:1–10
  1956b   A difference in mortality rate and incidence of kernicterus
            among premature infants allotted to two prophylactic antibac-
            terial regimens. Pediatrics 18:614–625
  1958   The influence of the thermal environment upon the survival of
            newly born premature infants. Pediatrics 22:876–886

Silverman WA
  1961   Dunham's Premature Infants, 3rd Ed. Hoeber, New York
  1966   Informed consent. Pediatrics 38:373–374
  1968   Oxygen therapy and retrolental fibroplasia. Sightsav Rev 38:
            131–134
  1969   Prematurity and retrolental fibroplasia. Sightsav Rev 39:42–
            46
  1977   The lesson of retrolental fibroplasia. Scientific American 236
            (No. 6):100–107
  1979   Incubator-baby side shows. Pediatrics 64:127–141

Singer P
  1976   "Bioethics": The case of the fetus. New York Review of
            Books, August 5, 1976

Smith CA and Kaplan E
  1942   Adjustment of blood oxygen levels in neonatal life. Am J Dis
            Child 64:843–859

Smith CA et al.
  1949   Adjustment of electrolytes and water following premature birth
          (with special reference to edema). Pediatrics 3:34–48

Smith CA
  1957   Reasons for delaying the feedings of premature infants. Ann
          Paediat Fenn 3:261–272

Smithells RW
  1975   Iatrogenic hazards and their effects. Postgrad Med J 15:39–52

Sounding Board
  1978   Clinical evaluation of Laetrile: Two perspectives. New Engl
          J Med 298:216–219

Speck WT and Rosenkranz HS
  1975   Potential genetic effects of phototherapy for neonatal jaun-
          dice. Proc Am Assoc Cancer Res 16:16

Spencer SM
  1955   Mystery of the blinded babies. Saturday Evening Post June
          11, 1955

Steinfels M O'B
  1978   New childbirth technology: A clash of values. Hastings Center
          Report XX:9–12

Stern L
  1975   Comment in Gellis SS: The Year Book of Pediatrics. Year
          Book, Chicago, p 25–26

Stevenson SS et al.
  1953   Some effects of exogenous thyroid or thyroxin upon premature
          infants. Pediatrics 12:263–271

St. Leger AS et al.
  1978   The anomaly that wouldn't go away. Lancet 2:1153

Stowens D
  1965   Hyaline membrane disease. Morbid anatomy, hypothesis of its
          pathogenesis, and suggested method of treatment. Am J Clin
          Path 44:259–270

Strang LB and McLeish MH
  1961   Ventilatory failure and right-to-left shunt in newborn infants
          with respiratory distress. Pediatrics 28:17–27

Strauss MB (ed)
  1968   Familiar Medical Quotations. Little Brown, Boston

Surgeon-General William H. Steward
  1966   Memorandum to heads of institutions conducting research with
            Public Health Service Grants, February 8, 1966

Szewczyk TS
  1951   Retrolental fibroplasia: Etiology and prophylaxis. A prelimi-
            nary report. Am J Ophth 34:1649–1650
  1952   Retrolental fibroplasia: Etiology and prophylaxis. Am J Ophth
            35:301–311
  1977   Quoted by United Press International: Protecting babies from
            blindness. East St. Louis, January 26, 1977

Tannenbaum AS and Cooke RA
  1977   Research involving children, in Appendix to Report and Rec-
            ommendations on Research involving Children of the National
            Commission for the Protection of Human Subjects . . . etc.
            DHEW publication No. (OS) 77-0005

Tauber I
  1958   The Population in Japan. Princeton University Press, Prince-
            ton, NJ

Taylor ES and Gordon HH
  1948   The premature infant program in Colorado. The Mother, Quart
            Bull Am Comm Nat Welfare 10:5–11

Terry TL
  1942   Extreme prematurity and fibroplastic overgrowth of persistent
            vascular sheath behind each crystalline lens. I. Preliminary
            report. Am J Ophth 25:203–204
  1945   Retrolental fibroplasia in premature infants. V. Further studies
            on fibroplastic overgrowth of persistent tunica vasculosa lentis.
            Arch Ophth 33:203–208

Townsend EH and Squire L
  1956   Treatment of atelectasis by thoracic traction. Pediatrics 17:
            250–257

Tuskegee Syphilis Study Ad Hoc Advisory Panel (Jay Katz, Chairman)

(undated)   Final report on charge three. Report to Doctor MK DuVal,
            HEW Asst. Secty. for Health and Scientific Affairs

United States Bureau of the Census
  1975   Statistical Abstracts of the United States, p 380

Unsworth AC
  1948   Retrolental fibroplasia; preliminary report. Arch Ophth 40: 341–346

Van Gelder DW
  1965   Magnesium sulfate enemas for respiratory distress syndrome (Letter and reply by Doctor Stowens). Pediatrics 35:355–356

Vengusamy S et al.
  1969   A controlled study of feeding gastrostomy in low birth weight infants. Pediatrics 43:815–820

Venn J
  1866   The Logic of Chance (An unaltered reprint of the third edition of this classic was made available as a "Fourth Edition" by Chelsea Publishing Co., NY, in 1962.)

von Fritz K
  1952   Relative and absolute values, in Anschen RN: Moral Principles in Action: Man's Ethical Imperative. Harper, New York

Wallace HM et al.
  1950   Prematurity as a public health problem. Am J Pub Health 40:41–47

Walster GW and Cleary TA
  1970   A proposal for a new editorial policy in the social sciences. Am Statistician 24:16–19

Warley MA and Gairdner D
  1962   Respiratory distress syndrome of the newborn—principles of treatment. Arch Dis Child 37:455–465

Watch Tower Bible Society and Tract Society of Pennsylvania

(undated)   Jehovah's Witnesses and the question of blood. Pamphlet

Webster C
  1976   The Great Instauration: Science, Medicine and Reform. 1626–1660. Holmes and Meier, NY

Wechsler H et al.
  1977   The Horizons of Health. Harvard University Press, Cambridge, MA

Wegman ME
    1977   Annual summary of vital statistics—1976. Pediatrics 60:797–804

Werner E et al.
    1967   Cumulative effect of perinatal complications and deprived environment on physical, intellectual, and social development of preschool children. Pediatrics 39:490–505
    1971   The Children of Kauai. University of Hawaii Press, Honolulu

Westin B
    1958   On the amount of gastric contents in the normal and the asphyxiated newborn infant. Acta Paediat 47:354–356

Whitehead AN
    1925   Science and the Modern World. Macmillan, New York

WHO Report
    1976   Health aspects of human rights. WHO Chronicle 30:347–359

Wilson JL et al.
    1942   Respiration of premature infants. Response to variations of oxygen and to increased carbon dioxide in inspired air. Am J Dis Child 63:1080–1085

Winckel F
    1882   Ueber Anwendung permanenter Baeder bei Neugeborenen. Centralblatt Gynäkologie 38:1–19

Yankauer A
    1955   Information memorandum New York State Health Department Feb. 17, 1955

Yankauer A et al.
    1956a   The rise and fall of retrolental fibroplasia in New York State. Preliminary report. NY State J Med 56:1474–1477
    1956b   Institutes for physicians and nurses in the care of premature infants: Evaluation of five years' experience. Pediatrics 18:95–101

Ylppö A
    1917   Uber Magenatmung beim Menschen. Biochem Zschr 78:273–293
    1954-55   Premature children: Should they fast or feed in the first days of life? Ann Paediat Fenn 1:99–104

Zacharias L
  1952   Retrolental fibroplasia: A survey. Am J Ophth 35:1426– 1454
Zuntz L
  1906   Die Sauerstofftherapie in der Geburtshilfe, in Michaelis M:
            Handbuch der Sauerstofftherapie. A Hirschwald, Berlin, p
            522

Index

Authors quoted by name in the text are listed in the index; those cited in Notes and References are listed in the bibliography section, alphabetically, under name and date. Abbreviations after page numbers: f=figure, t=table, fn=footnote, ap=appendix, n=notes.

a
b
c
d
e
f
g
0 h
1 i
8 2 j